FACE THE FACTS
THE TRUTH ABOUT FACIAL PLASTIC SURGERY
PROCEDURES THAT DO AND DON'T WORK

ANDREW A. JACONO, MD, FACS
FACIAL PLASTIC AND RECONSTRUCTIVE SURGEON

D1409111

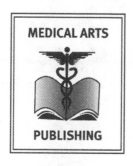

MEDICAL ARTS

PUBLISHING

This book is not intended to serve as a substitute for a physician, nor is it the author's intent to give medical advice contrary to that of an attending physician.

FIRST EDITION

Library of Congress Cataloging-in-Publication Data

Jacono, Dr. Andrew A.
        FACE THE FACTS The Truth About Facial Plastic Surgery Procedures That Do and Don't Work / Dr. Andrew A. Jacono — 1st ed.
                p.   cm.
        Includes index.
        ISBN 0-9779171-1-8
        ISBN-13 978-0-9779171-1-2
        1. Surgery, Plastic — Popular works.   2. Facelift — Popular works.
        3. Eyelid Lift — Popular works.   4. Botulinum Toxin — Therapeutic
        use — Popular works.   5. Skin — Wrinkles — Prevention.   I. Jacono, Andrew
        II. Title.

Library of Congress Control Number: 2006900459

To my wife Eva Jacono, my life partner;
to my children Andrew, Arianna, and Gavin,
whose smiles feed my soul; and to my patients,
who make it all worthwhile.

Contents

Acknowledgments

I would like to thank the many friends and colleagues who have assisted me in my development as a surgeon and/or in the creation of this book: my colleagues and friends at the New York Eye and Ear Infirmary; my colleagues and friends at the the North Shore University Hospital in Manhasset and the Long Island Jewish Hospital; Melody Lawrence and Georgette DeAndressi for reviewing the manuscript; Andrew Grivas for translating my ideas into descriptive yet creative illustrations; Doris Murray for her creative ideas and layout of the manuscript; Dr. Vito Quatela, my mentor; Dr. Paul Sabini for his friendship; Andrew Lerner, a good friend and positive supporter; my dedicated staff members Harriet, Patricia, Lou Ann, and Georgette.

And a special thanks to my patients for urging me to write this book.

Chapter 1
The Face is a Special Place.

Chapter 1
The Face is a Special Place.

Snake oil. What does snake oil have to do with facial wrinkles? Nothing at all, this is the point. Every day there are more and more products and surgical and non-surgical treatments available to improve the inevitable signs of aging – facial lines, wrinkles, and folds. The problem is that a vast majority of the skin care products and treatments do not deliver the changes we desire. It is not uncommon for us to spend hundreds sometimes thousands of dollars, and walk away without a discernable difference in our appearance.

We are living longer and more productive lives today than ever before. The average life span and life expectancy in the United States have grown dramatically in the last century, from 47 years in 1900 to 78 years in 1996. It is a natural extension of our expanded years that we want our appearance to reflect the health and vitality within us. Interestingly, the changes from cosmetic surgery can improve our health. Countless times I have seen patients change their approach to their physical well being after surgery due to the positive effect on their mind set. Again and again I see patients embrace a workout regimen, eat healthier and follow a skin care regimen after a procedure. This in turn motivates them to make more changes; it gives them the confidence to succeed at work and in their relationships. When you're performing at your peak mentally, physically and emotionally you're a better partner, parent, professional, lover, and friend.

According to the American Society of Plastic Surgeons over 9 million cosmetic procedures were performed in 2004. Last year the American Academy of Facial Plastic and Reconstructive Surgery noted that more and more women and men are undergoing facial rejuvenative procedures for facial lines, wrinkles, and folds. Men are buffing their image to excel in a competitive workplace. Less invasive treatments are becoming more popular as technology advances. Facelifts are performed through smaller incisions with less recovery time, risk and pain. The science of skin care has ascended to levels never imagined. Newer treatments including laser resurfacing, Restylane, Radiance and Botox therapy are reducing recovery to the time required for lunch. In fact most procedures, even major surgeries, are what I consider "lunchtime." They are performed as out-patient procedures in my office over a few hours. The medical advances that have made this possible are as follows:

Twilight Anesthesia allows patients to have procedures in a deeply relaxed state without the debilitating effects and risks of general anesthesia. Patients walk out of my office on their own an hour after surgery.

Endoscopic (telescopic) surgery technology allows me to perform forehead and facelifts with small incisions in the hairline using instruments the size of drinking straws. Essentially scarless surgery with a recovery time measured in days, not weeks.

Smaller and hidden incision surgery has allowed plastic surgeons to perform "stealth surgery." Shorter incision or "mini" facelifts have reduced incision lines to a third of what was used just 5 years ago. Eyelid lifts are often performed through incisions on the inside of the eyelid that are not visible at all.

Non-surgical techniques have allowed us superb results without going under the knife. Soft tissue fillers (Cosmoplast™, Restylane™, Captique™, Perlane™, and Radiesse™) and fat injections in the face can reduce folds; microdermabrasion, diamond peels, laser therapy and light chemical peels tighten the skin's surface and stimulate new collagen growth. Thread Lifts and Thermage™ treatments promise a non-surgical face lift.

Amongst this technologic revolution there is often a problem. I routinely hear from patients during consultations that they were sold a skin care system, or received a treatment at a spa, or with a dermatologist or plastic surgeon with little or no improvement. It is an investment of time and money, and the whole process can be very disappointing. Then there are those who are willing to take their quest to the next level and undergo a more invasive procedure. Maybe it is a Botox treatment, or an injection with the newest injectable filler for facial lines such as Restylane or

Radiesse. Sometimes it is a minimally invasive procedure such as a "Thread Lift" or Thermage™, or a more aggressive surgery (an eyelid lift or face lift). For some patients these more aggressive methods do not provide the desired result.

Why does this happen? There are two main reasons. First there are some treatments that are like snake oil and do not work. The second is that the wrong procedure was chosen for the problem, so that even if it was executed by the most skilled physician the problem is not fixed. Countless times I have consulted with patients who have had an eyelid lift that was performed perfectly, and yet they still have "crow's feet". This is because an eyelift is not the appropriate therapy for "crow's feet"!

The object of this book is to give you a crash course in facial plastic surgery, dermatology and skin care, and to demystify and define surgical and non-surgical cosmetic facial treatments for aging. It will give you the information you need to understand what it is that is contributing to your aging appearance, and will allow you to approach your doctor with confidence and gain the knowledge necessary to make an informed decision. Yes, there are different classes of facial folds, lines and wrinkles, and each is treated differently. I will use language and analogies that are easy to understand, as well as descriptive illustrations. There are many Before and After pictures of patients of mine who have so graciously given consent to being included in this book. The knowledge you gain will empower you. I have also included **Pearls of Wisdom** throughout the book to emphasize the key points that will help keep you on track.

Welcome to a wonderful journey, and I hope you use this book as a road map to reach your destiny. Now let's talk about you, and the changes you would like to make.

Chapter 2
The Skin and the Subsurface Framework: Understanding Aging Skin and the Aging Face

Chapter 2
The Skin and the Subsurface Framework:
Understanding Aging Skin and the Aging Face

Our skin is a living painting whose canvas represents the way we live our life. How do people see your painting? Does it convey a healthy lifestyle, or one that is replete with pollutants such as cigarette smoke and excessive sun exposure? We enter the world with smooth, supple flawless skin that can be transformed into the crepey, wrinkled, thin and sagging skin of middle age. This process occurs due to a host of different factors that we can control (how we treat our skin, our diet, whether we smoke or stay in the sun) and those that we cannot control (genetics, heredity, and gravity). Before we can understand how these factors affect our appearance we need to understand the science and structure of the skin and (what I like to call) the "subsurface framework" of the face. This will help us build the knowledge of how to rejuvenate our aging skin and our aging facial appearance.

The Skin

The skin is an organ, just like our heart, lungs, liver and kidneys. It performs a laundry list of vital functions; it is our body's first defense against infections from bacteria and viruses, it regulates temperature, and it is the sensor we use to negotiate the external world. Unlike our internal organs which are protected from the external world, our skin is like our armor and develops many flaws as it protects us.

Your skin consists of three basic layers, and each of these layers has its own intricate structure. The most superficial layer is the epidermis, the next deeper layer is the dermis, and the deepest layer is the fat layer *(Figure 1)*.

Epidermis. The surface layer of the epidermis is the *stratum corneum* and is composed of dead cells that protect our skin; it is truly like our armor. It helps retain our skin's moisture and oil. The *stratum corneum* is shed continuously and replaced with new cells from the deepest layer of the epidermis called the *basal cell layer*. The other cell type in the epidermis is the *melanocyte* that produces the color and pigmentation of the skin by producing a protein *melanin*. African Americans have the

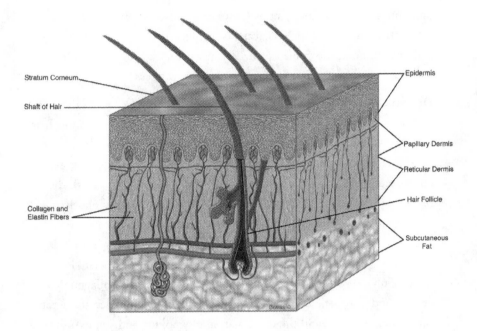

Figure 1.
The three layers of the skin include the superficial epidermis,
the middle dermis, and the deep fat. The dermis contains
most of the skin's collagen.

same number of melanocytes as Caucasians, however the melanin concentration in African Americans is higher. As we age, this layer becomes thinner, more disorganized causing the skin to feel and look rough and dry. Sun exposure accelerates this process.

Dermis. The dermis makes up about 80% of the thickness of the skin, and is its "workhorse" and heartbeat. It contains sebaceous glands, hair follicles, sweat glands, blood vessels and the nerve sensors which allow us to feel light touch, temperature, and pain. All these structures are enmeshed in a dense network of *collagen* and *elastin (elastic fibers)*, the primary proteins that support the skin, give it strength and elasticity. The dermis undergoes atrophy with age; elastic fibers degenerate reducing the resilience and elasticity of the skin, and collagen bulk is lost causing the skin to become thinner and allow surface wrinkles to form. Sun exposure causes *dermal elastosis* with further collagen degeneration and disorganization of elastic fibers. Smoking further accelerates the loss of collagen, and the combination of smoking and sun exposure is not additive but synergistic (greater than the sum of the two).

Fat Layer. Under the epidermis and dermis is tissue composed mostly of fibrous tissue and fat. Its function is to insulate the body and further protect the organs; it is a shock absorber of sorts. This helps keep the skin plump and smooth. Loss of fat as we age results in depressions in the skin, and causes the skin to sag and fold.

The Subsurface Framework of the Face

The skin of the face does not simply lie on top of the facial skeleton but is attached to it through a combination of deeper attachments to the bone. It is like the roadway of a suspension bridge; if we think of the roadway as the skin which is held up by the supporting cables or these deep tissue attachments. These deep tissue attachments include the *SMAS, platysma, periosteum* and the *osseocutaneous ligaments* of the face *(Figure 2)*. Their strength or lack of strength dramatically affects facial appearance irrespective of the quality of the skin. The skin can be perfectly smooth and supple and yet sag due to loss of its supporting cables.

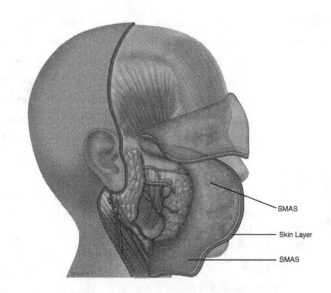

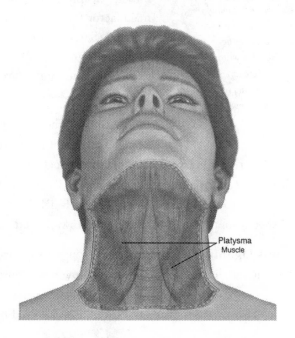

Figure 2.

*The deep facial muscle layers include the SMAS in the face
and the Platysma in the neck.*

SMAS. *SMAS* is an abbreviation for the superficial musculoaponeurotic system, and now you know why it is abbreviated. This is the layer underneath the skin and is a fanlike connective (or connecting) tissue layer that supports the full thickness of the skin we just described, the epidermis, dermis and fat layer. The *muscles of facial* expression are deep to the *SMAS*. The *SMAS* attaches the skin to the muscles of facial expression (the muscles that make us smile, frown and move our eyebrows, eyelids and cheeks).

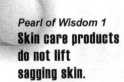

Pearl of Wisdom 1
Skin care products do not lift sagging skin.

If the skin is sagging, it sags as a result of weakening of deep muscular attachments. Applying creams to the surface of the skin will not penetrate to these layers, and will do nothing to reverse the aged appearance of the face.

The *SMAS* runs from the top of the head through the neck to the top of the chest. In the neck the *SMAS* continues as a layer that doctors call the *platysma*. As we age the attachment of this layer loosens with both the skin superficially and the facial muscles deeply causing it to sag. The main factor that causes this to occur is gravity. (Smoking weakens all tissue of the body and the *SMAS* is no exception, causing it to weaken before its time.)

Periosteum. The periosteum is the next deep layer of facial connective tissue. It is strong burlap like layer of tissue that connects the facial muscles to the skull. It is affected by gravity and smoking similar to the SMAS, and causes the full thickness of the face to droop off the facial skeleton with time. The periosteum supports the forehead, eyebrows, eyelids, and cheeks.

Osseocutaneous Ligaments. These are the strongest supporting cables of the skin. They attach directly from the skin, through the muscles to the facial skeleton. They are supportive mostly in the middle portion of the face and cheeks. This is another deep structure that is affected by gravity.

Muscles of Facial Expression. The muscles of facial expression are just underneath the *SMAS* layer, and are the deepest layer of the face. They animate the face, giving us the ability to smile and frown.

Chapter 3
Three Types of Facial Lines and Wrinkles

Chapter 3
Three Types of Facial Lines and Wrinkles

Yes, believe it or not all facial wrinkles are not created equal. They are different in three respects:

1) What causes them
2) Where on the face they exist
3) How they are best treated.

The chapter that preceded this one taught us the anatomy and science of the skin that will help us understand why one treatment works for one type of facial wrinkle, and not another. The three types of facial wrinkles are:

1) Wrinkles of motion
2) Wrinkles of surface damage, and
3) Wrinkles of sagging tissue.

TYPE 1: Wrinkles of Motion

We laugh, we frown, and we concentrate, and over time, those expressions leave their marks upon our face. The facial lines of motion are the direct result of contraction of delicate facial muscles underneath the skin surface. This causes the **overlying** skin that is attached by the *SMAS* (a deep connecting tissues layer, see Chapter 2) to the muscles of facial animation to wrinkle and fold. These wrinkles are unrelated to the health and youthful appearance of the skin! They become more obvious as we age because all three layers (the epidermis, dermis, and fat layers) of the skin become thinned and fold more easily with facial expressions.

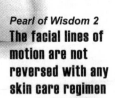

Pearl of Wisdom 2
The facial lines of motion are not reversed with any skin care regimen

because they are generated from the muscles deep underneath the skin. Creams and products applied to the skin do not penetrate this deep, and they do not stop these muscles from flexing. No matter what we apply to the skin surface it cannot affect this change, even if the product is excessively expensive.

The lines of facial motion are the wrinkles around the eyes ("crow's feet"), vertical lines between the eyebrows ("frown lines", what I like to call the "elevens"), and horizontal forehead wrinkles. The facial muscles that generate these changes are the muscles of facial expression and include the *orbicularis oculi* muscle for the "crow's feet", the *corrugator supercilli* for the "elevens", and the *frontalis* for the horizontal forehead lines *(Figure 3)*.

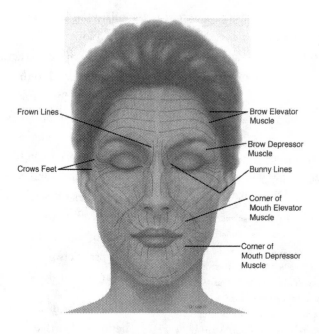

Figure 3. *Facial wrinkles that come from facial expressions include the crow's feet around the eyes, the horizontal forehead lines and the frown lines between the eyebrows.*

There are many devices that are sold to stimulate the facial muscles, strengthen them, and hence "tighten the face". Now that you are educated in the structure of the face you cannot be fooled by these marketing campaigns. Remember, sagging of facial tissues is related to thinning of the skin's *dermis* and weakening of the supporting *SMAS*, and *facial ligaments*. The muscles of facial expression are deep to these sagging tissues, and strengthening the muscles of facial expression will not affect the sagging overlying skin and SMAS. In fact, these products probably worsen the appearance of the skin over time.

Pearl of Wisdom 3
Flexing your facial muscles excessively will worsen your facial wrinkles.

Repeated flexing of the muscles, and folding the overlying skin over and over again, causes wear to the skin surface. Our skin is no different from an old leather coat that we have worn for many years. Repeated flexing of the elbows of the coat causes the leather's surface to get wrinkled and etched permanently. Contracting the underlying muscles of facial expression can similarly etch our skin surface causing the lines of surface damage, which are the second classification of facial wrinkles. Facial exercises and the Facial Muscle Stimulating Units (FMSUs) often sold on television at high prices are therefore a waste of time and money.

TYPE 2: Lines of Surface Damage

The lines of surface damage are the wrinkles etched in the skin itself, which are there even when the face is not moving and is static. Because they are within the skin, they are not related to sagging of the deeper underlying tissues that support the skin. These lines are like the texture of the fabric of a piece of clothing, for example the herringbone pattern in a wool jacket. No matter how you fold or pull the fabric, the pattern is unchanged.

The lines of surface damage are created by two forces – aging and thinning of the skin, and repeated motion of muscles of facial expression. As you recall from Chapter 2, with aging all three layers of the skin become thinner. This causes the skin to involute. These areas of involution have even more collagen loss, creating a line in the skin. The dermal layers in a wrinkle are thinner than the surrounding skin. The lines of surface damage can be anywhere on the skin of the face, head and neck. One of the more troubling areas where they occur is circumferentially around the lips. They are often called the "lipstick bleed lines" because lipstick will travel up these lines after it is applied. These are the lines we can prevent with the appropriate skin care that maintains dermal thickness. We can also accelerate these wrinkles before our time when we thin the layers of the skin with sun exposure and smoking.

The lines of facial motion, the winkles around the eyes ("crow's feet"), vertical lines between the eyebrows ("frown lines"), and horizontal forehead wrinkles, can become lines of surface damage over time. Just as we discussed earlier with the leather coat analogy, decades of motion generated by the facial muscles accelerate the wear of the skin surface in areas where it repeatedly folds; the folding causes loss of dermal collagen and elastin in the skin in areas that we recognize as wrinkles. As we will learn later, if we are proactive about preventing the face from flexing this way at an early age we can prevent surface damage.

Believe it or not physicians use a grading scale for the lines of surface damage called the Glogau Scale (created by Dr. Richard Glogau, University of California, San Francisco). The severity on this scale will often dictate the treatment as we will see later. The Glogau skin aging classification scheme is as follows:

- **Glogau 1- Mild (age 28-35 years)**
  Minimal to no discoloration or wrinkling, no keratoses (skin overgrowths), generally no need for foundation or makeup

- **Glogau 2 - Moderate (age 35-50 years)**
  Wrinkling as skin moves, slight lines near the eyes and mouth usually a need for some foundation

- **Glogau 3 - Advanced (age 50-60 years)**
  Visible wrinkles all the time, noticeable discolorations, visible keratoses, generally a need for heavy foundation

- **Glogau 4- Severe (age 65-70 years)**
  Severe wrinkling throughout, gravitational and dynamic forces affecting skin, yellow or gray color to skin, prior skin cancer, makeup not usable because it cakes and cracks

TYPE 3: Lines of Sagging Skin

The lines of sagging skin are a result of two factors working together – time and gravity. The longer we are alive, the more time gravity has to pull, albeit slowly, at the deep tissue supports or "cables" of the facial skin, i.e. the *SMAS, periosteum*, and the *osseocutaneous ligaments.* If we could live 2 hours of every day on our heads and 12 hours on our feet, our skin would not drop as much as we age.

Beyond external factors (smoking and a stressful lifestyle) genetics and familial predisposition will determine how quickly these cables weaken. I have had patients in their early 90s where these supports had weakened only to that of the average 60 year old; and I have had women and men in their thirties (and their parents and grandparents who preceded them) who looked 15 years older than their chronologic age because of their familial predisposition to early weakening of these supports.

There is a characteristic way that the lines of sagging tissue appear as we age with each decade. Just like gravity acts, we age from the top of the face down. The upper third of the face ages first, followed by the middle third of the face, and finally the lower third of the face and neck *(Figure 4)*. (There are, as always, familial variations on this concept.) Usually in our **mid to late thirties,** the supporting tissues of the eyebrows and the upper and lower eyelids weaken. This results in *brow ptosis* (a dropped brow) with heaviness and folded sagging skin between the eyebrows, hooding and folds in the upper eyelids, and bulging under the lower eyelids with grooving. In our **early to mid forties** the *malar fat pad* (cheek fat pat) descends resulting in the *nasolabial folds* (folds between the corner of the nose and corner of the mouth) and fuller face with loss of the width of the cheek bones. Finally in our **late forties to fifties** the lower third of the face drops. The *SMAS* and *platysma* weaken. The *marionette lines* (lines between the corner of the mouth and chin on either side) then form as the

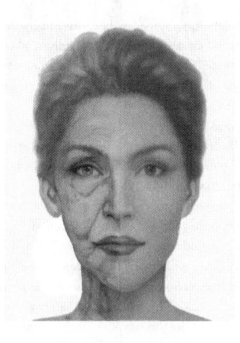

Figure 4.

Computer generated image of a woman's face.
Half represents her face in her late sixties and the
other half in her early thirties. Note how the
upper, middle and lower thirds of the face sag.

jowls cause loss of definition of the jaw line. Eventually the neck loosens causing excess skin and fat under the chin, a condition physicians actually call the *turkey gobbler* deformity. With further loosening of the *platysma* in the neck, vertical bands of tissue form between the chin and the lower neck called *platysmal bands*.

As aging continues, the degree of ptosis, or dropping of the deep facial tissue, increases. It can become so severe that the eyebrows and eyelids can droop in front of the eyes, blocking vision. The lower eyelid's supporting tissue can weaken until the lower eyelid turns outward, affecting our ability to close our eyes – making them excessively dry. The neck can drop until one can draw a straight line from the chin to the chest.

The lines of sagging skin are often best treated with more invasive surgical procedures as we will discuss later *(Before and After Patient 1)*. Other treatments are available that are less invasive such as Thread Lifting and ThermageTM, but tend to deliver a less dramatic result. Now that you understand the three types of facial wrinkles, you are ready to discuss the specific ways each group is best treated.

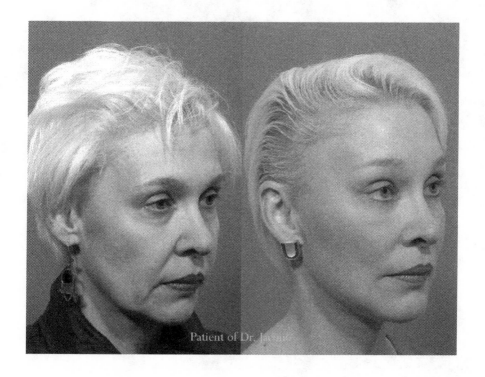

Before and After Patient 1.
Patient had a ScarFree Facelift,™ *neck lift, lower eyelid lift and*
chin augmentation.

Chapter 4.
Facial Wrinkles: The Lines of Facial Motion

Chapter 4.
Facial Wrinkles: The Lines of Facial Motion

As you recall the facial lines of motion are the direct result of contraction of delicate facial muscles underneath the skin surface. This causes the **overlying** skin that is attached to the facial muscles to wrinkle and fold. You do not have to be a facial plastic surgeon to realize the way they should be treated is to stop the muscles from contracting. This results in a flattening of the overlying skin. Hence the winkles around the eyes ("crow's feet"), vertical lines between the eyebrows ("frown lines", the "scowl", what I like to call the "elevens"), and the horizontal forehead wrinkles disappear *(Before and After Patient 2).*

Pearl of Wisdom 4
Treat your facial wrinkles when you are young.

Procedures that stop facial lines of motion are ones that I will suggest to many of my younger patients (in their 30s) who, by many people's standards, do not need them because their facial aging is just starting. These treatments are great as a preventative measure. As you remember from the previous chapter, the repeated contraction of the underlying muscles of facial expression can stretch our skin surface. I routinely inject my face with Botox to prevent the wrinkles on my skin surface before they occur. This treatment when combined with the appropriate skin care regimen (we will discuss skin care in Chapter 9) is our best defense against aging before it occurs.

There are **only two treatments** to stop the muscles from flexing. One is **Botox** injections, and the other is surgical manipulation of these muscles so that they can no longer fold the skin. There are benefits and disadvantages to each approach, but when executed well both methods produce fabulous results.

Botox Injections

"What, you expect me to put poison in my body?", is a comment I used to hear all the time 5 years ago. Now, with FDA approval, Botox injections are viewed by most in society to be no different than going to your local spa for a facial. During 2004, almost 3 million Botox procedures were performed. I think this is

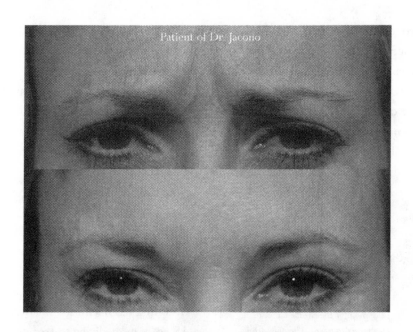

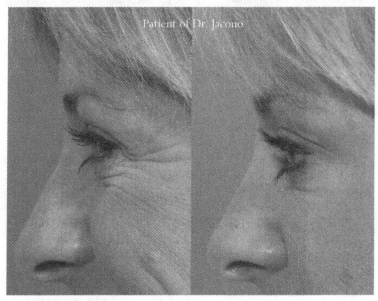

Before and After Patient 2.

Botox for frown lines (upper photograph) and crow's feet (lower photograph).

wonderful because the treatment results are impressive, it is easily tolerated, and it is one of those "lunchtime" treatments that can be done during the normal course of your workday. It is the most common injectable treatment that I administer in my practice. It is different from all the other injectable treatments, which fill crevices and lines in the face but do not stop motion in the face.

Botox is botulinum toxin, which comes from *clostridium botulinum*, a type of bacteria. It blocks the impulses that nerves send to muscles, paralyzing the muscles. Using a very fine needle, the surgeon injects the most active facial muscles – between the eyebrows, in the forehead, and around the eyes, as we described in Chapter 3. Botox has been used for over 15 years in medicine to treat spastic muscular disorders and is extremely safe. I have a friend who is a dermatologist who suffers from spinal muscle spasms. To treat his problem the quantity of Botox his doctor injects in his back is 16 times what we normally inject in the face. Even at these high doses there are no dangerous side effects.

After your injection you may not exercise or lie down for 4 hours, as this can make the medicine absorb unevenly or drift to places it was not intended to

Pearl of Wisdom 5
There is no free lunch when it comes to Botox treatments.

I have noticed that many patients will price shop for the cheapest Botox treatments in town. When physicians offer discounted Botox there is a reason. Botox is supplied to doctors in a powdered form, and before it can be injected it must be mixed with saline. The greater the amount of liquid that is mixed, not only the cheaper the Botox treatment, but the shorter period of time it lasts, because it is diluted. I have seen dozens of patients who have Botox last only 6 weeks, not 6 months. If you figure out the cost of maintaining the diluted result for 6 months with a doctor who charges less, it is twice what you would spend if you paid full price for a non-dilute treatment. The price should be your guide. $500 is the usual cost for a treatment that is not diluted.

go. It takes 72 hours before the effect starts to take place, and full penetration of the Botox can take up to 1 week. Sometimes a touch up may be necessary to even the result at 1 week. The result from Botox should be effective for four to six months. After the first treatment the muscles atrophy, similar to when a limb is in a cast and not used for six weeks. Because the muscles are weaker, I find that the second treatment after the first one has worn off tends to last 6 to 7 months. Complications are rare with Botox unless the medicine moves outside the target area. A droopy eyelid is a possible complication that lasts the length of the result (or maybe a little shorter) when the area over the eyebrows is treated. This is why physicians stress restrictions for the first 4 hours after treatment.

Botox can also be used to lift the eyebrows and the marionette lines, and smooth dropped neck skin. These affects are described in Chapter 6: Face Cocktails.

Muscle Motion Altering Surgery

The major drawback to Botox is its temporary effect, but there are more permanent, surgical ways of dealing with the wrinkles of facial motion. All of these procedures require that the muscle is interrupted (cut) surgically so it can no longer flex and have its effect on the overlying skin. As we discussed previously with respect to Botox

Pearl of Wisdom 6
The lipstick bleed lines that are around the lips cannot be treated with Botox.

The treatment is aggressively diluted so that it does not completely paralyze the muscles around the mouth, because if you did, even though the lip lines would be gone, you would not be able to speak, smile or kiss normally. There would be the risk of you looking like a stroke victim if your mouth did not move. From a common sense point of view, if the treatment is so diluted it does not affect much of a result. The bottom line here is save your money. These lines are surface wrinkles, and their treatment is addressed in the next chapter.

injections, you do not want to paralyze all facial motion and expression, as this would cause facial distortion and blunting.

There are minimally invasive surgeries to treat the scowl between the eyebrows and the crow's feet around the eyes. I will start by discussing the vertical lines (the "elevens") and the fullness between the eyebrows. As you remember from Chapter 3, the *corrugator supercilli* muscle is a horizontal muscle right above the eyebrows that, when contracting, causes the "elevens." This muscle can be cut without leaving any incision on the face. During an endoscopic browlift, through a few small incisions in the hairline, an endoscope can be passed down into this area releasing these muscles **(Before and After Patient 3).**

It is no different than the laparoscopic (telescopic) removal of a gallbladder that is so commonly used by surgeons today. This technique has only existed for about ten years in plastic surgery, but has been performed in this country on hundreds of thousands of patients. Due to its high technical nature all patients should interview their physician about the physician's experience with the procedure. Choosing a facial plastic surgeon can be a difficult task, and I hope I can help you with some good guidelines later in this book.

Pearl of Wisdom 7
An eyelid lift does not get rid of "crow's feet".

*"Crow's feet" traditionally have not been treated with surgical methods. I routinely see patients who were promised by a plastic surgeon that an eyelid lift to resuspend sagging eyelid tissue would correct their crow's feet. A standard eyelid lift will not accomplish this. There is a new procedure that has recently been described that is performed through an eyelid incision. The muscle around the eye, the **orbicularis oculi** muscle, is cut stopping the folding of the crow's feet. The only article in the medical literature to date reports only 16 patients, not enough of a track record to warrant a trip down this path yet. With more time, and more long term follow up with patients, this may become a viable alternative to Botox for the eyelid wrinkles of motion.*

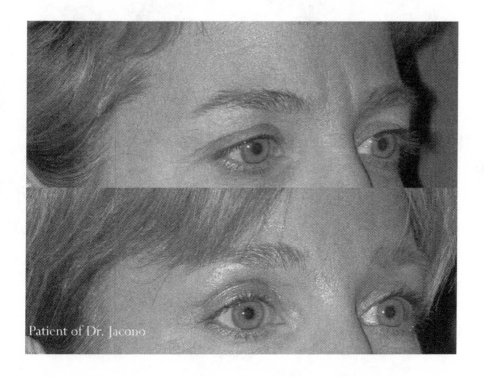

Before and After Patient 3.
Endoscopic brow lift with release of muscles creating frown lines.

Chapter 5.
Facial Wrinkles:
The Lines of Surface Damage,
Spackle and Sandpaper

Chapter 5.
Facial Wrinkles:
The Lines of Surface Damage, Spackle and Sandpaper

The best way to think of the way to treat the lines of surface damage is to think of how you would smooth the cracks and rough surface of an old wall in your home. As you run you hand along the wall you might notice some indented areas (similar to the wrinkles within the skin itself) and some raised rough areas (similar to the sun damaged roughened areas around the wrinkles). The solution for removing lines of surface damage in the face is just like the solution for repairing this wall – spackle and sandpaper. In facial plastic surgery the spackles are a variety of injectable soft tissue fillers (collagen, Cosmoplast™, Restylane™, Radiesse™, and Fat Injections to name a few). The sandpapers are resurfacing procedures such as chemical peels, laser resurfacing, and dermabrasion.

These are the two most effective treatments for more advanced damage to the skin surface. Skin care products can help to restore the skin significantly, but with more damaged skin the results can be less than what the doctor ordered. In a later chapter we will discuss the role and importance of skin care regimens and their relative efficacy. Generally speaking, they are wonderful for less damaged skin – Glogau 1 and lesser Glogau 2 type skin (see Chapter 3), and to treat aging before it occurs and help maintain results after surgery.

Resurfacing (Sanding) Procedures

Since the days of ancient Egypt, people have been using resurfacing methods to rejuvenate skin. The original chemical peel was lactic acid, an active ingredient of sour milk that was used topically by the nobles as part of an ancient skin rejuvenation regimen. In the Middle Ages, old wine with tartaric acid as its active ingredient was used for the same purpose. Today, these historical peeling solutions are known to contain alpha hydroxy acids (AHAs), which are the active ingredients responsible for the skin exfoliation.

Resurfacing procedures can be identified along a ladder of aggressivity, from superficial treatments, to medium depth treatments, to deep treatments. The difference between them has to do with the layer of the skin they cut through. Superficial treatments generally remove and resurface the epidermis, or top layer of the skin; medium depth treatments get down to the medium depth (half thickness) of the dermis, and the deep treatments get down into the deeper 2/3 of the dermis. The appropriate treatment is based on the depth of the wrinkle, or the layer of the skin the crevice extends into.

The three classifications of resurfacing procedures are chemical peels, laser resurfacing and dermabrasion. The major difference between these treatments is that chemical energy is used to polish the skin in a chemical peel, light/heat energy is used with lasers, and mechanical (sandpaper like) energy is used with dermabrasion.

Regardless of skin type, and regardless of the depth of resurfacing you choose, skin preparation is essential. Skin care is commenced 4 weeks pre-resurfacing. We will visit the issues of skin care in a later chapter dealing with Skin Care, Restoration, Maintenance and Prevention.

Pearl of Wisdom 8
Your skin color dictates what treatments are safe.

Not everyone is a candidate for every resurfacing procedure. Patients with darker skin are at risk for changes in their skin color with more aggressive treatments; the skin can either lighten (hypopigment) or darken (hyperpigment). Yes, as you already guessed, physicians have a classification of the darkness of skin and it is called the Fitzpatrick Scale (Dr. Richard Fitzpatrick, University of California, San Diego). This classification denotes 6 different skin types, skin colors, and reactions to sun exposure.

Type I (very white or freckled)
Always burn

Type II (white)
Usually burn

Type III (white to olive)
Sometimes burn

Type IV (brown)
Rarely burn

Type V (dark brown)
Very rarely burn

Type VI (black)
Never burn

People with Type IV skin or greater generally are at a higher risk for pigmentary disturbance after medium and deep resurfacing procedures. They are often better off sticking with more superficial treatments.

Superficial Resurfacing

Superficial resurfacing can be accomplished by all three methods.
Superficial resurfacing has the advantage of little or no down time, these
procedures are "lunchtime" and one can return to work after a treatment.
There can be some mild redness and irritation associated with them for a
day or two, however there are no raw surfaces to heal. These treatments are usually performed repeatedly over a short period of time, for example a chemical peel performed weekly for three months. The theory is that repeated resurfacing will not only remove the dead layers of cells from the epidermis, tighten pores and soften fine lines and wrinkles, but will stimulate collagen production in the dermis and tighten the surface. These treatments are generally safe for patients with dark skin types.

Pearl of Wisdom 9
Superficial resurfacing procedures can be classified as "snake oil" treatments if their ability to rejuvenate the skin is oversold.

Yes they can make some nice changes, but they are not a magic eraser. They will not remove lines like the more aggressive resurfacing treatments no matter how often they are repeated, and they cannot lift sagging skin and facial tissues like a lifting procedure (facelift, browlift, eyelid lift).

What follows is a listing of the three major classes of superficial resurfacing.

Alpha-(AHA) and Beta-(BHA) Hydroxy Acid Chemical Peels.
These acids are derived from fruit, milk, and other natural sources.
The most common of these is Glycolic Acid, which is derived from
sugar cane. They are very effective at turning over the skin's dead
surface layer, stimulating collagen production, and smoothing the
skin surface.

Microdermabrasion. This technique uses mechanical energy, with
small crystals being sprayed at the skin surface under pressure. A
vacuum sucks away the dead skin cells and crystals as it goes. The
pressure can be increased with repeated treatments to effect a better

result. This treatment, like all of its class, is "wash and wear." (It is very different from its distant relative that I call "macrodermabrasion" where a rotating abrasive brush gets to the medium to deep layers of the skin.)

"Light Touch" Lasers. These lasers are **non-ablative,** which means they do not melt the skin away with light and heat energy like their more aggressive counterparts that we will talk about later. These laser types (Nd:Yag, Alexandrite, and Pulsed Dye) will reorganize the collagen in the dermal layers of the skin, tighten it and give it a better texture. A Cool Touch version is available, where a cooling tip is used to minimize the discomfort during treatment.

Medium Depth Resurfacing

Medium Depth Resurfacing procedures include Trichloroacetic Acid (TCA) Peels, Laser Resurfacing and Macrodermabrasion. These procedures can get rid of the majority of the fine wrinkles in the skin completely, unlike a superficial resurfacing that results in these lines becoming softer. I often tell patients that medium depth resurfacing will get rid of about 60% of the lines. Since this type of procedure resurfaces to the mid dermal layer, it can remove the deeper wrinkles while causing the skin to tighten with the production of more collagen. Medium depth resurfacing will not tighten the skin to the degree that a lifting procedure would. This is because, as you remember, the reason the skin sags is that the deeper tissue attachments under the skin allows it to loosen. Because medium depth resurfacing results in a significant change in the tightness of the skin, it is an alternative to a lift in a patient who is starting to notice early jowling around the jaw line and sagging of the eyelid skin (usually a patient in their early 40s). We will spend a lot of time in the next chapter defining how surgery can provide a better result for the wrinkles of sagging skin.

Medium depth resurfacing procedures have a greater risk of complications than the superficial peels, but are extremely safe when used on the correct skin type by a skilled plastic surgeon or dermatologist. Patients with Fitzpatrick Class IV skin (darker complexions that tan easily) and higher can have pigmentary changes in the skin, including lightening and darkening of different areas, so patients with this skin type are generally not good candidates. Scarring is another possible adverse outcome, but when these procedures are performed at the appropriate energy settings, and at the appropriate depths of peeling and dermabrasion, the risk is extremely low.

Unlike superficial resurfacing treatments, these procedures can be painful when performed while you are awake. Local anesthetic injections to numb the skin surface, or twilight anesthesia, where you are dosing, are the ways I keep patients comfortable.

All deeper resurfacing procedures except Fraxel™ laser require that you take anti-herpes simplex virus treatment before and during the recovery phase as there is a risk of the chicken pox virus reactivating and causing ulcers. Which in turn can cause scarring while healing. As always an ounce of prevention is worth a pound of cure. What follows is a listing of the three major classes of medium depth resurfacing.

Trichloroacetic Acid (TCA) Peels. TCA peels can be administered in 20%, 30%, 35% and 40%, and as the percentage increases the depth of the peel increases. At lower concentrations it can be applied with the use of a local anesthetic to numb the skin, and with higher concentrations I believe it is better to have a "twilight" anesthesia where you are not awake, but not under the effects of general anesthesia. This is the type we might get in a dentist's office or during a colonoscopy. With a TCA peel is applied, there is no pain or burning past the application of the solution. Moisturizing ointments are applied for the ensuing week, and after about four days the dead skin surface peels off, almost the way old paint flakes off a wall. One week after the procedure all the skin has peeled leaving very smooth, new pink skin that almost looks like you have had a sunburn. This pinkness fades over the ensuing 3 weeks; camouflaging makeup can be applied one week after a peel.

Carbon Dioxide (CO_2) and Erbium/YAG Laser Resurfacing.
Unlike the superficial light touch lasers, these are **ablative** lasers that remove the skin layers by vaporizing or melting the skin. Removal of the medium depth with a laser encourages the growth of healthy new

cells. The thermal effect of the **CO₂** laser on collagen causes the skin to tighten a little more than with TCA peels. The **Erbium / YAG** laser is most commonly used for fine lines and wrinkles. It is a less aggressive laser than the **CO₂** laser, and uses a different wavelength of light that causes less thermal injury. The heat energy causes collagen contraction and new collagen formation in the dermal layers of the skin. The improvement seen with deeper wrinkles is not as good as with the **CO₂** laser, even at the same depth of penetration. The advantage to the Erbium/YAG laser over the **CO₂** laser is its lower risk of scarring and lightening of the skin's color. These effects have been reported to happen in as high as 7 % of patients, in some articles in the medical literature. After all medium depth laser resurfacing, an occlusive dressing is applied and not removed for 5 days. The dressing allows the skin to regenerate and heal over the surface. As with medium depth chemical peels all raw surfaces are healed over at 7 days and the skin remains pink for the ensuing 3 weeks.

Fraxel™ Laser. The Fraxel™ laser is a glass fiber laser that produces thousands of tiny but deep columns of treatment in your skin known as "microthermal zones". These zones penetrate the dermis (middle layer of the skin) but leaves the stratum corneum (top protective layer of the skin) intact. It has the advantage of no recovery time and the ability to be used on all skin types. A series of 4 to 6 treatments is necessary, spaced 1 to 2 weeks apart. Fraxel™ reduces facial wrinkles similar to but less than some of the more aggressive lasers we discussed above (CO2 and Erbium/YAG Laser) that require a 1 week recovery. Currently it is only FDA approved for eyelid wrinkles, but is being used by physicians for full facial treatments.

Macrodermabrasion. Macrodermabrasion produces a medium depth result, removing lines, wrinkles, acne scarring and raised hypertrophic (overgrown) scars. This is very different from microdermabrasion which is more like a loofah sponge for the skin, exfoliating and removing only the surface layer *(epidermis)* of the skin. Unlike a chemical peel that uses chemical energy, or a laser resurfacing that uses heat energy, dermabrasion is the process of *mechanically* removing the damaged layers of skin. In a lot of ways a macrodermabraded area is no different than a scraped knee when we were children. Usually a rotating brush or diamond wheel is used to penetrate into the depth of the skin in a graduated fashion. Because it is extremely dependent on the skill of the surgeon, it can be viewed almost as an art, with the physician sculpting the skin. Each line and wrinkle can be treated individually, with a lesser penetration for more shallow wrinkles, and a greater penetration for deep lines, Macrodermabrasion is wonderful for the deeper lines, especially those that radiate around the lips, the so called "lipstick bleed lines" *(Before and After Patient 4).* In fact, when used to penetrate more deeply it can be considered a deep resurfacing procedure. The healing face is the same as the others in the medium depth class. An occlusive dressing is worn, as in laser resurfacing; however the skin surface tends to weep, draining fluid for the first few days.

Deep Depth Resurfacing

The most aggressive way to resurface the skin is with a phenol peel. As we discussed above, a macrodermabrasion can also be performed to this level of depth. Since these two procedures resurface to the deep dermal layer, called the reticular dermis, they can remove the deepest wrinkles while causing the skin to tighten with the production of more collagen. These resurfacing methods are used on patients classified as severe in the Glogau Scale we noted above. Due to the aggressivity of deep resurfacing there are greater risks of scarring and hypopigmentation, or skin whitening. (Have you ever noticed how much the skin of older Hollywood celebrities can appear translucent, and pale, yet line free? This is the appearance of an individual who has had multiple deeper resurfacings.) The initial healing phase for these procedures is much longer, approximately 2 weeks, and the pink tone to the skin can last up to 3 months. As we have already discussed macrodermabrasion above, we will focus our attention here on phenol peeling.

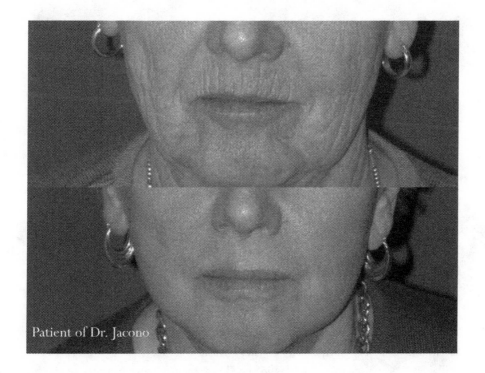

Patient of Dr. Jacono

Before and After Patient 4.
Dermabrasion for lipstick bleed lines. This patient also had a face and neck lift at the same time to treat her jowls and sagging neck.

Phenol Peels. Phenol produces the most dramatic results and is the most effective peeling agent currently used. The phenol produces a new zone of collagen that is thicker than that produced by laser or macro-demabrasion. The toxicity of phenol may be significant, and the procedure should be performed only by a physician who regularly performs this aggressive treatment. Phenol is absorbed through the skin, metabolized by the liver, and subsequently excreted by the kidneys. Overdoses may injure the liver and kidney and may lead to heart problems. For this reason, phenol peels should always be performed in an operating room, with a *board certified anesthesiologist* present. Surgery accomplishes more dramatic and long lasting results by re-establishing the supports, and removing excess sagging skin and tissue.

Wrinkle Filling (Spackling) Procedures

Soft tissue fillers are the spackle that fill the facial lines and creases, and they come in a large variety. Some are temporary, lasting 4 to 6 months, and some are permanent. These fillers are generally injected into the dermal layer of the skin, as this is where we lose collagen; it is the loss of collagen that causes the wrinkles in the skin to arise. You can think of these soft tissue fillers as replenishing the dermal layers of the skin. Where there is loss of the fat that underlies the skin, resulting in folds, these fillers can plump out sunken areas of the face or add fullness to the cheeks or lips. Common folds to be filled include the grooves between the corner of the mouth and nose called the nasolabial folds and the marionette lines between the corner of the mouth and the chin *(Before and After Patient 5)* The results of these procedures are often dramatic, and can refresh the appearance without more invasive surgical procedures.

The two major classifications of soft tissue fillers are those that are temporary and those that are permanent. Regardless of the treatment the discomfort associated with the injections can be minimized by applying a topical anesthetic cream thirty minutes prior to treatment. When lips and more sensitive areas are to be injected, local anesthetic is injected into a nearby nerve causing the whole are to become numb. This is called a nerve block. Although it requires an injection it makes the treatment that follows for the next ten to fifteen minutes painless. We will now review each of these treatments and discuss the risks and benefits of each.

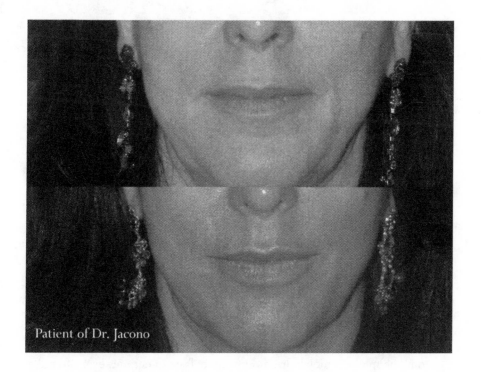

Patient of Dr. Jacono

Before and After Patient 5.
Restylane™ for nasolabial folds between the corner of the
nose and mouth. This patient aslo had her lips augmented with
Restylane™

Temporary Fillers

Temporary fillers are biologic implants, usually proteins, that are gradually reabsorbed by the body after they are injected. Our body recognizes them as foreign and thus gets rid of them. The most commonly used temporary fillers are **Collagen, Cymetra™/AlloDerm** (Human Dermis), **Restylane™** (hyaluronic acid), and **Radiesse™** (Hydroxyapetite or bone like minerals). Some of the fillers we have just listed are **not** FDA approved, but are safe when used by a physician who has experience using them.

Collagen is an older treatment for injecting facial lines, and has been used for almost thirty years, and yes, it is FDA approved. The traditional form of collagen comes from cows and is called Bovine. Because it comes from a different species, 3 percent of people are allergic to it. This means you must be skin tested twice (the testing process takes 1 month) so that you do not have a swollen face if you are allergic and it is injected. Collagen usually lasts 3 months, however some people will metabolize it extremely fast, sometimes even after 1 month. (There has never been a reported case of mad cow disease (bovine spongiform encephalopathy) from a collagen treatment, and there will not likely be one as the collagen is taken from closed herds in an isolated California ranch.) In 2003, the company that produces bovine collagen (Allergan) produced **CosmoDerm™** and **CosmoPlast™**, made of human collagen, that has been purified from human skin grown under controlled laboratory conditions. Because it is of human origin it requires no skin test, and this is its major advantage. It lasts the same period of time as bovine collagen.

Cymetra is particularized *dermis* (the middle layer of the skin) obtained from human cadavers. It replaces dermal losses that cause wrinkles with all the proteins that exist in the dermis, unlike collagen which is only one of the proteins in the dermis. The tissue is processed and all cells are removed to prevent transmission of any viruses or bacteria; the tissue is tested for hepatitis as well as the HIV virus. It is extremely safe and has been used in millions of patients without any reported transmission of any infectious disease. It is injected in the same way as collagen, and lasts about the same amount of time.

Restylane™ and Captique™ are non-animal stabilized hyaluronic acid (HA) and are among the newest of wrinkle-reducing fillers. Hyaluronic acid is another type of protein, like collagen, and is grown in a lab, but not obtained from human cadavers. It has been used for years in Europe, and has been approved by the FDA. **Perlane™** is also hyaluronic acid, just in a denser form. No skin test is required for these treatments. Recent studies have revealed that results after injections with hyaluronic acid are superior at 6 months when compared to collagen treatments. The repair is more durable but still temporary.

Radiesse™ is another of this long list of temporary fillers, and is not FDA approved. Radiesse is made up of microscopic calcium particles (hydroxylapatite) that are found in bone and suspended in gel. This is a safe material (one that is already in use for dental reconstruction, bone growth, and vocal cord injection) and one that has proven to be very compatible with the body. Unlike Collagen it does not require an allergy test, and studies show that it will last approximately 2 years, and can last up to five years, so it is more like a permanent filler. In rare cases a patient may experience tiny calcium deposits that may rise to the surface of the skin and appear like small white bumps that will disappear over time.

Sculptra™ is an enduring treatment approved by the FDA for restoration and/or correction of the signs of facial fat loss, or **lipoatrophy**. It is poly-l-lactic acid, a biodegradeable polymer. It is approved for use in people with human immunodeficiency virus, but cosmetic surgeons are using it for facial aging. Facial fat loss, or lipoatrophy, is the loss of fat beneath the skin, which can result in sunken cheeks, indentations, and hollow eyes. Sculptra® is a safe, synthetic, and biocompatible material that is injected below the surface of the skin in the area of fat loss. It provides a gradual and significant increase in skin thickness, improving the appearance of folds and sunken areas. It is not useful for more superficial lines and folds. No skin testing is required. Sculptra® has been safely used outside the United States since 1999 in over 150,000 patients under the trade names New-Fill™ and Sculptra™.

Permanent Fillers

The most commonly used permanent fillers are, **Artefill, Silicone**, and **Autologous Fat** (fat from our own body).

Artefill or Artecoll is a mixture of synthetic beads of plexiglass (polymethylmthacrylate) mixed with collagen. It has been used in Europe, but has not received FDA approval. After the collagen component dissipates, these beads permanently fill the wrinkles injected. **Silicone** is another synthetic liquid injectable filler that is not FDA approved. It has been injected into wrinkles and facial scars for over 30 years.

Autologous Fat does not have this inherit problem. Autologous simply means "your own", and since your own fat is transferred from one part of your body to another there are no real side effects. Using a thin cannula, or straw like tube, and light suction, fat is harvested from the abdomen, hips or buttocks. The fat must be harvested with specialized equipment, processed and washed with saline, and injected with the correct caliper needles. Why all this preparation? The reason is that

Pearl of Wisdom 10
The greatest drawback to Silicone, Artefill and Artecoll is that the body can react against these synthetic materials

and patients can experience local skin irritation and inflammation that will not go away. This does not happen commonly. The only way to get rid of the reaction is to cut it out, and this can leave permanent scarring. There are physicians who dedicate their practices to injecting silicone, and they are the best to administer these treatments due to their large volume of experience.

if you simply use a high powered suction and inject it without processing it, and inject it through any needle, the fat cells are not likely to persist past a few months. Fat cells are extremely fragile, and proper care is necessary to ensure that the injected fat will last permanently. After 1 year approximately 60 to 70% of what is injected lasts and stays with you permanently. For this reason more than you want is injected initially, and the problem is overcorrected. Quiz your doctor about how he or she performs fat transfers. Fat is globular and thick and cannot be injected into fine surface lines as it would make them look lumpy. It is best used to treat deeper folds to plump them out, for example the laugh lines around the corners of the mouth. The major drawback here is that you cannot simply open a package as you can with the other materials; this requires a surgical procedure.

Whether temporary or permanent, fillers cannot resuspend facial tissues that have fallen due to the effects of gravity. Chapter 7 will highlight all the procedures that help treat the lines, wrinkles and folds of the face that result from sagging skin.

Chapter 6.
The Face Cocktail

Chapter 6.
The Face Cocktail

Although this frothy title might suggest an intoxicating mixed drink for a patient who has undergone the knife, these elixirs are not alcoholic. This cocktail is a combination of injectable treatments, some of which have been discussed in Chapters 4 and 5, which when performed at the same time can provide extremely rejuvenating results. They represent a gentler alternative to a face lift by using plumping fillers and Botox. Although their results are temporary and not as dramatic as a face lift, injection cocktails are sufficient for patients in their 30s, 40s and 50s. It is important to use a combination of fillers at the same time, as different fillers (Restylane, Radiesse, and Cosmpolast) treat different surface wrinkles and folds depending upon their depth *(Table 1)*.

One of the important components of the Facial Cocktail, is the use of Botox to lift portions of the face. You have already learned in Chapter 4 that Botox is a neurotoxin that relaxes muscles, and is effective in relaxing the scowl lines between the eyebrows, the crow's feet around the eyes and horizontal forehead wrinkles; it can also lift facial sections including the eyebrows, the corner of the mouth/marionette lines (lines from the corner of the mouth to the chin) and neck bands.

The way to understand how Botox lifts the face is to understand that there is a constant tug of war going on in any section of the face. There are muscles that lift a portion of the face (for example the eyebrow) and opposing muscles that pull it down. If we inject Botox in the muscle that pulls things down, the muscle that lifts wins, and the result is that that portion of the face is lifted *(Figure 5, page 49)*. In this example the eyebrows are elevated creating a non-surgical brow lift. This also works when injecting Botox into the muscles that pull the corner of the mouth down, causing the marionette lines to flatten as the muscles that lift this area work unopposed. Another place where Botox is used is on the paired

Facial Cocktail Component	What Is It	How It Works	How Long It Lasts
Botox Cosmetic™	Neurotoxin that relaxes facial muscles.	Relaxes facial muscles removing crow's feet, frown lines and forehead lines. Will relax the muscles that pull the eyebrows down and corners of the mouth down giving these areas a lift. Relaxes neck bands that are dropped neck muscles	4 to 6 Months
Restylane™, Captique™, Hylaform™ or Perlane™	Hyaluronic acid a protein.	Fills facial wrinkles and folds such as the marionette lines, folds between the corner of the nose and the mouth. Can be used to fill grooves under the eyes, creating a non-surgical eyelid lift.	4 to 6 Months
Radiesse™	Calcium Hydroxyapatite, a mineral suspended in a gel.	Used in the deepest of facial folds, more substantive than Restylane.	9 to 12 Months
Sculptra™	Poly.-L-Lactic Acid a biodegradeable polymer.	Fills facial hollows that occur with facial fat loss with age.	12 to 18 Months
Cosmoplast™	Human Collagen	Used in superficial lines in thin skin where Restylane and Radiesse cannot be used.	3 Months

Table 1.

Guide to Facial Cocktail Injections to Rejuvenate the Face.

vertical bands in the neck that run from the chin to the chest. These bands are the platysma muscle of the neck, and they are apparent because this muscle pulls down when it is tensed. Generally speaking, a 40-50% improvement is obtained with the lifting affects of Botox.

The cocktail is the result of combining these lifting Botox injections with facial fillers *(Before and After Patient 6)*. We have learned in Chapter 5 that fillers are like spackle, they fill in lines. The type of injectable that is used is dependent upon how deep the lines are. Cosmoplast is best used in very superficial lines, Restylane™ is used for deeper lines and folds like those between the corner of the nose and mouth and the lipstick bleed lines around the lips. Radiesse™ is used for very deep facial folds that need more volume and a substantial augmentation. Radiesse™ and Sculptra™ are also great for bulking cheeks that have lost volume with age and sag. (Fat transfers are a more permanent way of accomplishing the same effect.) No one facial filler can be used on all wrinkles; for example if you inject Radiesse™ in the superficial lines it will leave white bumps in the skin. This is why often we will use a Face Cocktail, with Radiesse™ in one section, Restylane™ in another, and Botox to lift.

The whipped cream on the facial cocktail is a non-surgical eyelid lift with Restylane™. As we age the bags and grooves develop under the eyes that look like dark circles. The deep grooves under the eyes can be filled with Restylane™, causing the grooved areas to flatten and rejuvenating the eyes.

It is easy to see that a face cocktail that lifts the eyebrows, marionette lines, and neck, and fills in grooves under the eyelids, plumps cheeks, and fills in lines around the mouth and facial folds creates a face lift in a syringe that can easily knock 10 years off our appearance without surgery.

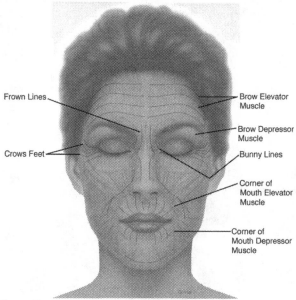

Frown Lines

Crows Feet

Brow Elevator
Muscle

Brow Depressor
Muscle

Bunny Lines

Corner of
Mouth Elevator
Muscle

Corner of
Mouth Depressor
Muscle

Figure 5.
Facial cocktails that use Botox injections can lift the eyebrows and the corners of the mouth (early jowls) by relaxing the facial muscles that pull them down.

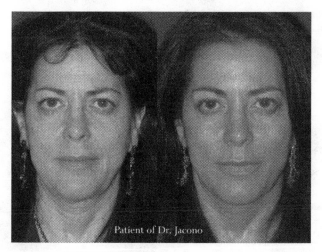

Patient of Dr. Jacono

Before and After Patient 6.
Facial Cocktail. Botox was used for frown lines and for a non-surgical brow lift. Restylane™ fills in the smile lines and augments the lips.

Chapter 7:
Facial Wrinkles: The Lines of Sagging Skin

Chapter 7:
Facial Wrinkles: The Lines of Sagging Skin

The wrinkles of sagging skin are those that result from loss of the deep tissue supports of the skin If you remember our analogy of the suspension bridge with the road representing the skin and the supporting cables representing the deep tissue supports of the skin, it is weakening of the cables that allows our facial roadway to buckle. In the face, weakening of the supporting cables leads to the following folds in the face that are characteristic of aging: upper and lower eyelid grooves, the folds underneath the dropped eyebrows, the nasolabial folds (between the nose and the corner of the mouth), the marionette lines (between the corner of the mouth and the chin), the jowls, the "turkey gobbler" neck, and the platysmal bands (vertical neck bands). In this instance plastic surgery is *not* "rocket science." If something has dropped due to loss of supports (cables) then you lift it. There are **non-invasive** and **invasive surgical** ways of approaching the problem. Surgery accomplishes more dramatic and long lasting results by re-establishing the supports, and removing excess sagging skin and tissue. No amount of creams, injections, or laser treatments will reverse sagging tissue, so save your money!

The aging process of sagging does not happen in isolation, and often those with sagging eyelids and jowls will have a significant amount of skin surface damage. Remember, our skin surface is like the fabric of our clothes, even when we stretch the fabric it's inherit pattern will remain, and so will etched lines in the surface of the skin after any lifting surgery. Wrinkles of surface damage have to be treated with resurfacing as we discussed in the previous chapter. Often these two different classes of procedures are combined; the eyelids are lifted to remove excess bags under the eyes and tighten the muscle, at the same time as a laser resurfacing is performed to remove the eyelid crow's feet. Let's take it a step further. If we really want to eradicate any and all lines within the skin, after we polish the skin with a laser we will paralyze the muscles around the eyes with Botox. This will prevent the lines of motion that occur as the muscles around the eyes contract when we smile, and by so doing prevent the skin surface from getting etched by the repeated folding of the skin.

This will improve the longevity of any resurfacing procedure.

All lifting procedures should last about ten years. That is without continued abuse of the skin – smoking, lying in the sun and drinking alcohol excessively. In these situations it will probably last more like 5 years. The face will continue to age slowly due to the effects of age and gravity. The good news is that the face still looks better at ten years than it did the day before the patient walked into surgery.

Obviously, there are ways of preventing these and all changes of the facial appearance from occurring (we will visit these in the next chapter), but our task in this chapter is to describe the procedures that lift the face, both the non-invasive and invasive surgical treatments. There are Six Pearls of Wisdom that follow, and if you understand them they will help you choose the appropriate procedure for your face, even if your doctor suggests otherwise.

Non-Invasive Lifting Procedures

There are two classes of non-invasive treatments to lift sagging skin. One is called **Thermage**™ which is a type of radiofrequency tissue tightening, and the other is called a **Thread Lift**, the most common of which are the Aptos Threads™.

Thermage

Thermage™ is a procedure that employs a radiofrequency (RF) technology that heats up the collagen in the deeper layers of the skin itself. This heating causes the collagen to tighten and remodel over time. The energy is applied to the skin surface with a handpiece, and there are no incisions or surgery required. There is no downtime, and the treatment takes up to 1 hour depending upon the amount of the face that is treated. This creates a healthier and smoother skin that is more youthful in appearance. The full result can take up to 6 months to evolve, with a gradual tightening to the collagen in the skin.

This treatment has been studied only in small objective trials published in the medical literature and the jury is out as to the degree of improvement expected and its longevity. One trial with 24 patients studied the effect of Thermage on brow lifting and showed the results were not uniform in all patients and that patient satisfaction was low *(Otolaryngology Head and Neck Surgery April 2004 Issue)*. Another study of 20 patients looking at how the middle and lower face tightens after this treatment revealed that patients had much better results if they underwent two treatments, and that after two treatments the overall change noted by both patients and physicians was modest *(Archives of Facial Plastic Surgery December 2004 Issue)*. In other studies, only 50% of patients experience noticeable improvements.

These measured results are quite different from the way the treatment is marketed by many physicians who offer it. Most patients are not happy spending upwards of $6000 on two treatments and getting a "modest" result.

Thread Lifts

There is now a less invasive procedure where threads with cogs or barbs are placed under the skin and tugged to suspend and lift the sagging tissue. Areas that are treated include the brow, dropped cheeks, jawline and neck. Two or three threads are placed in problem areas to recontour *(Figure 6)*. The procedure can be performed under local anesthesia. Theoretically collagen bunches around the threads causing an even further lifting effect.

Pearl of Wisdom 11
Thermage only lifts the face moderately at best.

If you understand the chapter on the skin and subsurface framework you understand that the deep tissue attachments and muscles under the skin droop and weaken with age; Thermage only treats the skin. It does not tighten these deep supportive tissues and therefore it cannot achieve dramatic tissue tightening as it only treats a small portion of the problem. In my practice I have performed many face lifts on patients who were oversold the effectiveness of Thermage. In my view it is most appropriate in one of three categories of patients:

1) Those who are just starting to age and are too young for a more invasive procedure in their thirties to early forties;

2) Those who are not looking for more than a subtle change (not someone with heavy jowls); and

3) Those who cannot have surgery due to health problems.

Due to the low patient satisfaction rate I do not perform this procedure in my practice, but refer appropriate candidates to physicians I trust who perform it regularly.

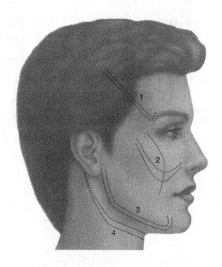

Figure 6.
Thread Lifts. *Four different locations for placement of threads under the skin to lift problem areas.*

Candidates should not have a lot of lax skin. Ideal candidates are those who have had a prior face lift, or those in their late 30s early 40s who have just started to have facial drooping. There are no long term studies that have documented the effectiveness or longevity of this procedure. In my experience this procedure lasts at most 12 months to 1 1/2 years.

I educate my patients about this fact as it is a big investment. At $500 per thread, and a treatment requiring 6 to 12 threads, it can cost $3,000 - $6,000 for around a one year result!

Pearl of Wisdom 12
Your face is like steak.

In thread lifting, although the threads are permanent, the tension placed on the deep tissues causes the threads to pull through our facial tissues over time. The face then sags again. Just like if you put a strong thread through a piece of steak and pull, the thread would not break, but over time, the thread would pull through the meat. Unfortunately, our facial deep tissues are no different than meat. Some new manufacturers are producing threads that have the ability to be tightened over time to maintain the result longer. The problem is that the threads are no longer in the same place after they release and pull through, so re-tightening them will not have the same effect.

Invasive Lifting Procedures

Surgery accomplishes more dramatic and long lasting results by reestablishing the supports, and removing excess sagging skin and tissue.

Upper Eyelid Wrinkles and Hooding, and Lower Eyelid Wrinkles and Grooves.

The eyes are the windows to the soul, however their outward appearance can project a tired look even when we feel vibrant and energetic. Their appearance will often invoke unwanted comments such as "have you been getting enough sleep" or "is everything alright, you don't look well." Both the upper and lower eyelids can contribute to this look *(Before and After Patient 7 & 8)*.

Upper eyelid skin becomes redundant as we age, and this causes "hooding" of the upper eyelids and loss of the natural upper eyelid crease. Sometimes this will prevent women from being able to apply makeup to the

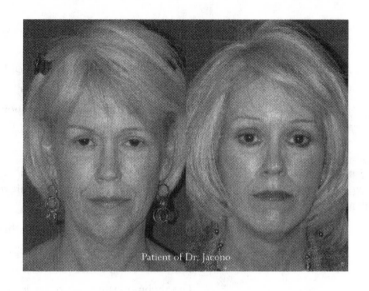

Before and After Patient 7.
Upper and lower eyelid lift. This patient also had an endoscopic browlift and ScarFree Facelift™ (See Chapter 8).

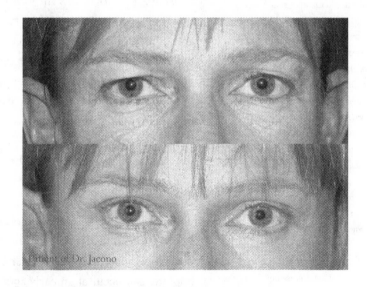

Before and After Patient 8.
Upper and lower eyelid lift

upper eyelids, and sometime it is so severe that it blocks vision. This can happen at a very early age as there are familial patterns of aging; I have performed upper eyelid surgery in women as young as thirty years old. These patients will tell me they started noticing the changes in their twenties and that everyone in their family has the same upper eyelid appearance.

Pearl of Wisdom 13
Many times patients need a browlift not an upper eyelid lift.

When the eyebrows drop they fall in front of the eyelids like a window curtain. You can do as much work as you like on the window (eyelids) but if the window curtain (eyebrows and brow skin) is blocking the window you will never see the work on the window. I see about 6 patients a month who had their upper eyelid lifted by another plastic surgeon but still have a heavy tired appearance of the upper eyelids. When I examine these patients the upper eyelid lift was executed perfectly. Unfortunately, a browlift was in order and not an upper eyelid lift. In some of these patients an upper eyelid lift and a browlift should be executed at the same time to give the best result. The best way to decide for yourself is to sit in front of the mirror and lift the eyebrows. If you like what you see, you do not need an upper eyelid lift.

An upper eyelid lift, or upper blepharoplasty, is one of the quickest recoveries amongst all cosmetic surgeries. It is often a patient's first facial surgery; it is socially acceptable, and the recovery time is 3 to 5 days. The techniques we use today have evolved to where the incisions are small and hidden in the natural curvatures so that they are nearly invisible. I perform this surgery with a local anesthetic injection and a twilight anesthetic. The incision is placed about ten millimeters above the upper eyelash line in the natural crease of the upper eyelid. Through this incision excess fat bags are removed and the excess skin is trimmed away.

Lower eyelid grooves are the result of excess fat under the eyes causing "bags" that leave shadowed grooves underneath. Excess saggy and crepey lower eyelid skin also contributes to this appearance. This, like upper eyelid hooding can occur at an early age along familial patterns.

The lower eyelid lift is performed with the same kind of anesthetic as with the upper lids, and often lower and upper eyelid surgery will be performed at the same time. There are two ways to perform a lower eyelid lift; one requires an external incision in the skin and the other is **incision-less**. The approach that is chosen is dependent upon whether excess skin needs to be removed or just the fat bags under the eyes. The external incision technique is used when extra skin needs to be removed, and the incision is placed just underneath (2 millimeters below) the lower eyelash line. This gives access to the lower eyelid's excessive muscle and fat, as well as allowing the skin to be trimmed and tightened. The incison-less technique (called a transconjunctival blepharoplasty) places an incision inside the eyelid, through the lining of the eye (the conjunctiva) to access the redundant muscle and fat. This technique is used on younger patients who have not yet developed excess skin. Sometimes a chemical peel or laser resurfacing will tighten the surface of the skin when combined with an incision-less lower eyelid lift.

Forehead Grooves, Dropped Brows, and Upper Eyelid Heaviness

The deep furrows and wrinkles of the forehead, the vertical scowl lines between the eyebrows, sagging eyebrows and heaviness on the upper eyelids all start in our mid thirties. You may recall that these furrows can be treated well with Botox injections, as they are lines of motion, but this treatment is temporary. A procedure

Pearl of Wisdom 14
Deep grooving below the eyelid bulge is not reversed with a lower eyelid lift.

This is another area where there is a high rate of patient dissatisfaction after cosmetic surgery. The deep groove under the eye is really the bone of the orbital rim (eye socket). If you touch this groove you will feel that the bone is directly underneath the skin, and there is no soft tissue or cheek pad overlying this bone. As you remember from Chapter 3, the malar fat pad, or cheek fat pad that overlies the cheek bones and this orbital bone drops as we age, this is called midface drooping. If a lower eyelid lift is performed, it removes the bags under the eye; however it accentuates this groove and can make the lower eyelids look hollowed out. To best rejuvenate this area a combination of a lower eyelid lift and a midface lift to lift the dropped cheek fat pad are best to accomplish a complete rejuvenation. We will discuss midface lifting later in Chapter 8: The ScarFree Facelift™.

called a brow or forehead lift is a more permanent way to remove these furrows; additionally it lifts the sagging brows and heaviness on the upper eyelids, something that Botox injections cannot accomplish *(Before and After Patient 9)*.

Browlift surgery has "come a long way, baby." The traditional browlift is performed through an incision that runs across the top of the head, from one ear to the other. This is a long incision and the invasive nature of this procedure results in prominent scarring, bruising and swelling, and a longer recovery. Side effects include numbness of the scalp (it feels like there is a permanent cap of numbness on the top of the head), hair loss along this large incision line, and the eyebrows often are in too high a position, giving what I like to call the "deer in the headlights" or startled/surprised look. A majority of plastic surgeons still perform browlifts in this traditional way, but there is a more advanced and less invasive way of accomplishing the desired result.

An endoscopic browlift, I believe, is the more appropriate way to accomplish the goals of forehead lifting surgery. Endoscopic simply means "telescopic". The surgery is performed through a few small incisions in the hairline, with a telescope the size of a drinking straw, and specialized instruments. It is the same concept as telescopic gallbladder excision: years ago when doctors removed your gallbladder they made an incision that was a foot long under the rib cage, and now with a few small incisions and a telescope the same surgery is performed with a quicker recovery and less scarring.

The endoscopic browlift is performed under twilight anesthesia. Through small incisions the forehead including the skin muscle is lifted off the bone *(Figure 9, page 74)*. The layer that attaches the overlying tissues to the bone is the periosteum. This burlap like layer is the one that weakens as you get older and allows the tissues to drop – it is one of the supporting cables that weakens. The eyebrows are detached from the orbital (eye socket) bone, so they can be lifted, and the corrugator muscle that causes the clefting between the eyebrows is cut. The tissues are then lifted and held into their elevated position with sutures.

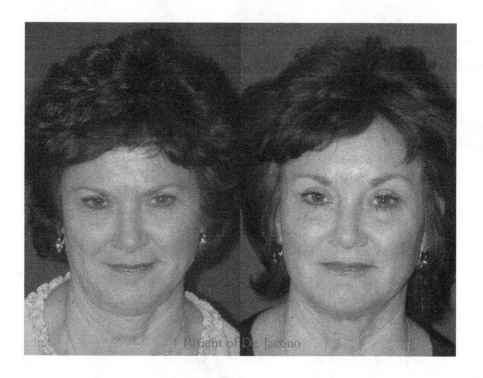

Before and After Patient 9.
Endoscopic brow lift.

An endoscopic browlift has an extremely quick recovery phase. The recovery time is usually 5 to 7 days. All incisions are in the hair line, so they are not visible to anyone. Common aspects of recovery include bruising around the eyes, and a sensation of numbness in the forehead that lasts from several weeks to several months.

Nasolabial Folds and Wrinkles, Sagging Cheeks, and Deep Lower Eyelid Grooves

All three of these changes are related to the descent of the midface malar fat pad as we discussed above. As gravity acts upon our face, it weakens the deep tissue attachments of the malar fat pad, and the periosteum, which allows the soft tissues to fall off the bone. The best way to understand the midface is to look at the face on profile, and draw a line from the top of the ear canal to the corner of the mouth. Everything above this line to the lower eyelid is considered the **midface,** everything below this line is the lower face and neck. This midface area is best treated with a procedure called the **ScarFree Facelift™** which is an endoscopic procedure to lift the dropped cheeks and will be discussed in Chapter 8.

Jowls, Marionette Lines, and Neck Wrinkles

As you recall from Chapter 3, the changes in the lower third of the face and neck occur due to loosening and sagging of the SMAS deep muscular layer in the face, and the *platysma* muscle layer in the neck. The skin in these areas also becomes redundant over time. This results in the jowls that create marionette lines, or wrinkles between the corner of the mouth and the chin; a blunting of the jaw line; a "turkey gobbler" in the neck; and vertical banding in the neck *(Before and After Patient 10).*

These changes are best corrected with a *rhytidectomy*, or facelift. A facelift best corrects the area below a line drawn from the ear canal to the corner of the mouth on profile view of the face. This is what I like to refer to as the lower face. There are three ways to perform a facelift; a traditional facelift, a mini facelift, and a weekend facelift. Each has its advantages and disadvantages, and not everyone is a candidate for all three procedures. It is the surgeon's job to inform you which treatment is best, and what results you can expect.

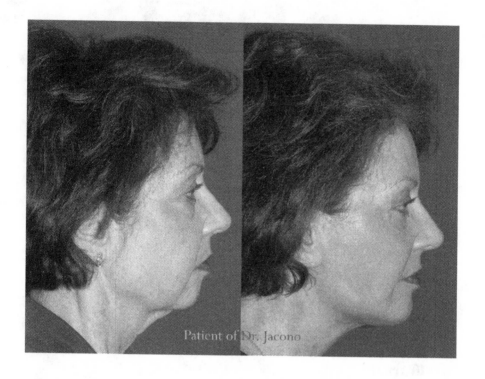

Patient of Dr. Jacono

Before and After Patient 10.

Face and neck lift with hidden incision. This patient also had a lower eyelid lift.

A traditional facelift is a two layer facelift, where the skin and the underlying SMAS are tightened separately during the procedure. (Years ago only the skin was tightened; in old Hollywood movies this gave the stars a "windblown" appearance.) The incision begins just below the sideburn. It travels down behind the tragus, the small knob of flesh in front of the ear canal, beneath the earlobe, then travels behind the ear, up three quarters the length of the ear and into the back of the hairline *(Figure 7)*. The skin is elevated off the face, the SMAS is elevated off the face, the extra skin and SMAS is removed, and the face is sutured back together.

At the same time many surgeons will perform a neck lift. A small incision is made under the chin, extra fat is removed that contributes to the

Pearl of Wisdom 15
Quiz your plastic surgeon as to how he/she places his/her facelift incisions (Figure 7).

Now that you have been educated on how an appropriate incision should be placed, ask your surgeon how he/she performs his/hers. The majority of plastic surgeons start with their incision in the hair on the side of the head above the sideburn. This is a problem because as the skin is pulled tight, and excess skin is discarded, a large amount of hair on the side of the head is removed. This leads to a very unnatural look called temporal (side of the head) alopecia (balding). Next time you are at the hair salon, look around at all the women with wet hair who are pulling their hair forward to cover the loss of hair on the sides of the head. The incision continues in front of the ear leaving a visible scar. This limits your hairstyle choices. I have a funny story about this issue in my office. I have an employee who worked at Bergdorf-Goodman in Manhattan as a sales representative before she began working for me. On her first day of work she asked me why "all the high society women I took care of looked like aliens with no hair on the sides of their head." The reason, as you now know, is because they had had surgeons who made this classic error – one that can be completely avoided. Another issue is that the limb of the incision behind the ear should be on the back of the ear itself, not on the skin where the ear and the neck meet, and should curve 2/3 of the way up the ear. Why is this so important? The reason is that as we age the skin continues to fall, and if the incision is not placed on the back surface of the ear it will drop with more age and gravity, leaving an obvious scar lower in the neck, usually 5 to 10 years after surgery. This scar is extremely difficult to hide and can be quite embarrassing.

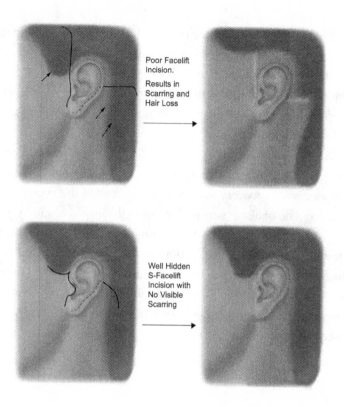

Poor Facelift
Incision.

Results in
Scarring and
Hair Loss

Well Hidden
S-Facelift
Incision with
No Visible
Scarring

Figure 7.

Poor face lift incision versus well placed hidden incision. Poor incision placement in the upper diagrams results in visible scars and hair loss.

"turkey gobbler", and the *platysma muscle* is tightened (the muscle that separates in the center causing vertical bands in the neck). It is important to lift the face and neck simultaneously. It is advantageous as there is only a small hidden incision. Additionally the appearance of the neck is one of the telltale signs of aging; when the neck lift is not performed the face on the neck looks like the wrong lid on a jar.

The initial healing face of a traditional facelift takes 7 to 10 days, and I usually suggest that patients give themselves two weeks out of circulation . Common aspects of recovery include bruising around the eyes, and swelling in the cheeks. The bruising gets pulled down through the skin by gravity and often will settle around the chest. The most common complication from a traditional facelift is a collections of blood under the skin, or *hematoma*, and this must be evacuated as it can compromise the viability of the skin. It happens in about 1 % of patients. Infections are extremely rare in facelift surgery, and must be addressed immediately. All patients experience numbness in the face for 6 weeks to 3 months in the area where

Pearl of Wisdom 16
A Traditional Facelift does NOT lift the Midface/Cheeks.

I cannot stress how important it is to understand this concept. I see many patients in consultation who want a total facial rejuvenation, and I explain how they will need both a midface lift and a traditional facelift (or a variant of a traditional facelift such as the mini or weekend facelift we will describe below) to accomplish their goals. Then they go to visit another plastic surgeon for an opinion, where , he/she explains that a midface lift is not required because he/she is going to perform a "total facelift" and this will lift the midface as well. This is an absolutely false. The reason they will tell a patient this is few doctors perform a midface lift. Rather than lose a patient, they try to sell a traditional facelift as something it is not. This fact is true not because I say so; dozens of clinical trials have proved that the traditional facelift approach does not accomplish lifting of the midface.

the skin was elevated. Initially this will be a blessing as there is little pain; after a few weeks it is a nuisance, and you just want your face to feel normal.

There are two serious possible complications of face lifting. One is the possibility of damage to the facial nerve (the nerve that moves the face) damage, but this is extremely rare (less than 1 %) in experienced hands. Most times nerve weakness is temporary as nerves get stretched during surgery, and will regain normal function over 3 to 6 months. The other serious complication is skin death. This can occur due to a hematoma as we stated previously, but more commonly happens to smokers. The nicotine in cigarettes makes the blood vessels in the skin constrict, and therefore the blood supply to the skin is less than normal after surgery. Where skin is lost, there is a growth of scar tissue which can be unsightly and require revisional surgery at a later date. For smokers the risk of skin death is 14 times that of non-smokers, and all smokers should stop for two weeks before and two weeks after surgery. Nicotine gums have the same affect on the skin as smoking so they also should be avoided.

The **mini-facelift** is another way to rejuvenate the lower third of the face, and is also called a short scar facelift, or an S-Lift. It is called an S-lift because the shape of the small incision used is that of an S. It starts at the top of the ear, runs in front of the ear like the traditional facelift, and ends just behind the earlobe without running into the scalp **(Figure 7, page 65).** The skin is elevated as in a traditional facelift, but unlike a traditional facelift the SMAS is not elevated off the face, but is simply pulled and tightened with stitches. This reduces the amount of bleeding, and of swelling from surgical trauma, and quickens recovery. The results are probably not as long lasting as a traditional facelift. A neck lift is usually performed in combination as with a traditional facelift. The risks are similar to those of a traditional facelift, but the risk of nerve injury is significantly less because the SMAS is not as aggressively lifted.

The **weekend facelift** is not a facelift at all but a combination of a submental (or neck) liposuction and a specialized chin implant *(Before and After Patient 11)*. The chin implant is one that augments the jaw line in the area just before the jowl that is dented inward, called the pre-jowl. The implant fills out the pre-jowl region and camouflages the jowl. It is placed through the same small incision under the chin used for a neck lift. The liposuction in the neck removes the extra fat of the "turkey gobbler", and as the area heals the skin scars upward slightly reducing the amount of hanging skin. However, since extra skin is not removed the liposuction will decompress the fat, often allowing the skin to hang a bit. This looks better than an extremely full neck, but it does not accomplish what a facelift can. This is a great procedure for patients with early jowl and neck changes in the forties, and the recovery is literally 3 to 5 days. There are fewer risks, but amongst the more concerning are the possibility of chin implant infection and rejection (rare — less than 1%) and facial nerve injury (less than 1 %).

Pearl of Wisdom 17
Facial liposuction does not improve jowling.

I have seen dozens of patients in consultation after a facial liposuction who are unhappy. They were sold a facial liposuction to collapse the jowls by another surgeon, underwent the procedure, and were left with little improvement. Patients are attracted to facial liposuction because it is cheaper than a facelift and has a quicker recovery time. Unfortunately liposuction in the face will decompress the jowls, allow them to hang more loose skin, and it often leaves depressions in the overlying skin. Liposuction is much better suited to the neck. The point here is save your money if more severe jowling is your primary concern.

Mesotherapy is an alternative to liposuction in the face. Mesotherapy is an injection of a chemical called phosphatidylcholine/deoxycholate that helps dissolve and treat localized fat deposits. Although there are some studies that show mesotherapy helps dissolve fat cells in test tube conditions, its safety and efficacy in contouring facial fat deposits has not been proven. For this reason liposuction is still the best and most reliable choice.

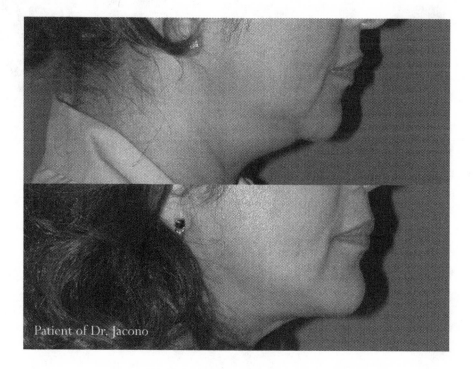

Patient of Dr. Jacono

Before and After Patient 11.

The weekend face lift is simply a neck liposuction and a specialized chin augmentation. A patient can recover from this procedure over a weekend.

Chapter 8.
The ScarFree Facelift™

Chapter 8.
The ScarFree Facelift™

The midface, the area where the nasolabial folds, and the sagging cheeks occur, is a very special place in facial plastic surgery. It is an area that for the past fifty years in cosmetic surgery was ignored and was very poorly treated. As you recall, we age from the top down, so that while the brows and eyelids start to change in our thirties, the midface begins to drop in our forties *(Before and After Patients 12 & 13)*.

All these changes are related to the descent of the midface cheek/ malar fat pad as we discussed above. As gravity acts upon our face, it weakens the deep tissue attachments of the malar fat pad, which allows the soft tissues to fall off the bone. The best way to understand the midface is to look at the face on profile, and draw a line from the top of the ear canal to the corner of the mouth. Everything above this line to the lower eyelid is considered the midface, everything below this line is the lower face and neck *(Figure 8)*.

A **midface lift** is truly the forties and early fifties facelift. Midface lifting has been performed by a small group of plastic surgeons for the past 8 years, and now is gaining recognition in the popular media. As a result there are a lot of doctors who are beginning to *learn* this procedure on their patients.

There are two ways to perform a midface lift. One way is through two incisions, one underneath the eyelashes, similar to that used in a lower eyelid lift, and the other through the mouth above the upper teeth. The tissues including the muscle, fat and skin are elevated off of the facial bones in the midface and cheek, and elevated to a higher place. Deep suspension sutures are used to hold it up. The major problem with this approach is that there is a high rate of malposition of the lower eyelid; the weight of the cheek tissue tends to pull the lower eyelid downward and outward. This is called *ectropion* and its high rate of occurrence with this approach has been well documented in the plastic surgical literature. It results in a very unnatural and distorted, wide eyed appearance, that also makes the eyelids appear droopy.

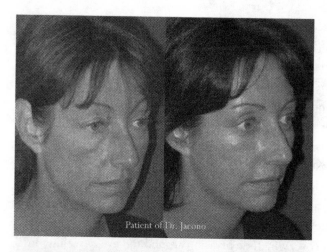

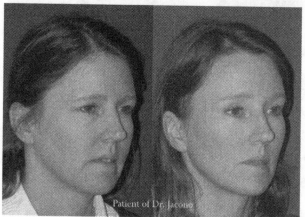

Before and After Patient 12 & 13.

Two examples of a ScarFree Facelift™ to lift dropped cheeks and brows. Both patients also had a lower eyelid lift.

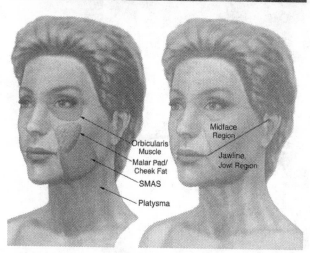

Orbicularis Muscle
Malar Pad/ Cheek Fat
SMAS
Platysma
Midface Region
Jawline, Jowl Region

Figure 8.

A line drawn from the ear to the corner of the mouth separates the midface from the remainder of the face. The midface begins dropping in the early forties and is best treated with a ScarFree Facelift™.

The other approach to midface lifting is through four slit like incisions, hidden in the hairline. This is called a ScarFree Facelift™ *(Figure 9).* The dissection is continued downward past the brows, and underneath the malar fat pad over the surface of the central facial skeleton. This approach is technically very demanding, and requires specialized telescopic equipment. Since the suspension is approached from above, there is no lower eyelid malposition; in fact this procedure lends more support to the eyelid, making it tighter against the eye.

The initial healing face of the ScarFree Facelift™ takes 3 to 5 days, and I usually suggest that patients give themselves 7 days out of circulation. All incisions are in the hair line, so that they are not visible to anyone. Common aspects of recovery include bruising around the eyes, swelling in the cheeks, and a slight pulling at the outer corners of the eyes giving the eyes a more almond shape. The change of the shape of the eyes is temporary, and releases after a few weeks. The only serious risk with this procedure is the possibility of damage to the facial nerve (the nerve that moves the face), but this is extremely rare (less than 1 %) in experienced hands.

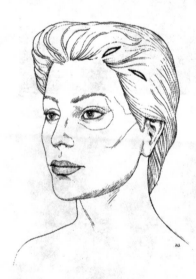

Figure 9.
ScarFree Facelift™ incisions hidden in the scalp hair. This procedure lifts dropped cheeks. These same incisions are used for an endoscopic browlift.

Chapter 9.
The Truth About Skin Care Products, Wrinkle Prevention, and Sunscreens

Chapter 9.
The Truth About Skin Care Products, Wrinkle Prevention, and Sunscreens

We have already reviewed the structure of the skin in Chapter 2 and the changes that occur with aging in all three layers of the skin – the epidermis, the dermis and the fat layers. The old cliché states that "an ounce of prevention is worth a pound of cure, and in skin aging nothing could be more true. While we do not have control over our genetic tendency toward skin aging, there are environmental factors that accelerate the aging of the skin and there are things we can do through skin care that can reverse even our genetic predisposition. When we take active steps to prevent aging of the skin by avoidance and by supplementing and building the skin through skin care, many of the surgical procedures can be avoided completely. We are specifically speaking of the wrinkles that occur within the skin itself, the "lines of surface damage", as we already know that wrinkles related to sagging skin and wrinkles of motion are the result of deeper tissue components.

Be aware that in the skin care realm, there is a lot of "snake oil." If you cruise any department store, pharmacy, or day spa counter, you will be astonished by all the claims on all the beautifully packaged skin care products. Eye creams, wrinkle creams, exfoliants and moisturizers abound, and they can be extremely expensive! I remember there was a time when I was still in medical school when my wife spent $300 a month on skin care. The problem here is that the majority of skin care products sold over the counter are ineffective, and do little more than moisturize. Even if they have good active ingredients, the concentration of these ingredients is dilute. The reason is that higher concentrations of these good active ingredients can only be sold with a prescription from a physician. Generally speaking if ingredient X is good for your skin, you will not get enough of X in the cleansers and creams at your favorite skin care store.

This is not to say that prescriptive skin care dispensed by a physician always works well to diminish the signs of aging, including sagging of skin and facial wrinkles. I have consulted with hundreds of patients who have been prescribed a dozen different physician strength skin care products with no success. There is a small group of skin care products that have definitively proven to improve facial wrinkles in prospective, randomized, double blinded studies. Without this rigorous research, the effectiveness of skin care products is anecdotal at best.

The object of this chapter will be to demystify skin care treatments. We will focus on the best ways to prevent aging of your skin, treat the wrinkles you already have, and maintain the results of different cosmetic procedures you may undergo to improve your appearance.

Wrinkle Prevention

There are three ways to prevent aging of the skin:

1) Avoiding **skin pollutants/wrinkle generators,**
2) Protecting the skin from daily sun exposure, and
3) Supplementing and nourishing the skin with prescriptive skin care that helps maintain the skin's supple and smooth appearance.

There are four major **Wrinkle Generators** – sun exposure, smoking, excessive alcohol intake and poor nutrition. **Sun exposure** used to be thought of as extremely healthy 30 years ago; many people may remember applying baby oil/iodine mixtures to the skin to magnify its intensity. Sunlight helps maintain our bodies' levels of vitamin D, an important nutrient to the body. What we later learned was that all this sun exposure resulted in an increasing rate of skin cancers decades later – today the number of newly reported cases is greater than it has ever been in human history. If this is not enough, premature aging of the skin is another side effect. Sun exposure causes build up of dead cells in the superficial *epidermal* layer of the skin, giving it the appearance of leather in the most sun damaged individuals. It also causes *solar elastosis*, a process where the collagen and elastin molecules in the deeper *dermis* of the skin become disorganized and thinned. These changes in the dermis are the direct cause of thinning of the skin, and wrinkle formation within the skin.

If even this is not enough, sun exposure causes the production of terrible molecules called **free radicals** in the skin. Our skin cells use oxygen to produce energy, and sunlight causes this oxygen to turn into free radicals that can damage virtually every part of a cell including its DNA.

In fact these scavenging particles are believed to be the major culprit with respect to aging, heart disease, and cancer. Our body produces these as part of normal functioning, but sunlight accentuates their production. There are antioxidants that we can use to prevent the damage free radicals may cause to our skin, both by improving our nutrition and by their application to our skin. We will discuss the ways to use antioxidants to our advantage later in this chapter when we talk about skin care and maintenance.

Smoking and Alcohol use are another two important pollutants of the skin. Smoking has multiple affects on the skin. First the nicotine in cigarettes causes the blood vessels in the skin to constrict, and reduces blood supply to the skin which deprives the skin of nourishment. As you recall from the previous chapter, this reduced blood supply to the skin can cause the skin to die after a facelift. Chronic malnourishment causes all layers of the skin to thin and involute, loss of collagen and elastin, and the formation of wrinkles. It also causes the release of more free radicals. Excessive alcohol use causes malnourishment of many essential vitamins and nutrients in our body including the B vitamin complex and folate that are essential to skin cell reproduction and health. Of course like most vices, it too causes free radical production to increase in our blood stream. This obviously does not mean that a glass of wine with dinner is out of the question; in fact we have all heard of the benefits of consumption of red wine in moderation with respect to heart disease.

Malnourishment either as a result of a fast-food diet, or from chronic dieting or excessive alcohol intake decreases the concentration of many antioxidant vitamins in our body. Repeated fluctuations in weight as the result of failed diets in turn repeatedly expands and deflates the skin, resulting in skin that sags more and has more wrinkles. In today's environment it is extremely rare for people to have such severe malnutrition that they deplete their body of essential trace minerals, and of vitamins, except in the case of alcoholism.

Sun Blocks and Skin Protection

Aside from avoiding wrinkle generators, we need to protect our skin in everyday life from the sun to prevent photoaging. Photoaging is the term for long-term thinning, sagging and wrinkling that is caused by sunlight. The difference between skin that is photo-aged and that which is just plain aged is the difference between the skin on the face and hands versus the skin on the buttocks. Sunlight contains two kinds of ultraviolet (UV) light – longer UVA rays and shorter UVB rays. UVB is the main cause of sunburn and most skin cancers. UVA, while not as powerful as UVB, penetrates more deeply in the skin and is the chief culprit behind skin wrinkling and leathering.

The American Academy of Dermatology recommends that a sunscreen or sunblock with an SPF of at least 15 be applied about a half hour before you go outside each day. SPF stands for Sun Protection Factor, and measures protection against sunburn-creating UVB (but not damaging UVA). If it normally takes five minutes to get a sunburn on a summer day, a product with an SPF rating of 30 would let you stay outside 15 times longer (75 minutes). They also recommend a SPF of at least 30 if you will be out in the sun for more than an hour. Sunblocks that contain zinc oxide and titanium dioxide block UVA rays that cause facial wrinkling; others, without these two essential ingredients, do not.

Antioxidants may also offer protection to the skin and prevent skin aging while nourishing and supplementing its deeper layers. This is a new frontier in skin care, and studies of the efficacy of anti-oxidants are lacking. The major antioxidants in the skin are Vitamin C and E which we get from our diet, and coenzyme Q10, glutathione and lipoic acid, which are produced by our bodies. There is also a synthetic antioxidant used in skin care products called idebenone. As you remember from above, free radicals cause chronic damage to the cells of the skin, and antioxidants can neutralize these dangerous molecules. Increasing these antioxidants with supplemental pills can replenish our natural reservoir, but you need very large amounts and you get only a modest effect; there are mechanisms in the body that control how much of the anti-oxidants are absorbed, and how much can eventually be delivered to your skin.

Applying these antioxidants directly to the skin is one way of solving the problem of getting additional antioxidants into the skin. These antioxidants are inherently unstable compounds, and their ultimate delivery into the skin in topical preparations can be questionable.

Even without this evidence I do suggest that patients increase their oral intake of antioxidant vitamins, and use **Topical Vitamin C Therapy.** Vitamin C is **Ascorbic Acid** and is essential for the production of collagen, the strong connective tissue that holds the skin together. Collagen is the skin's glue. Centuries ago, when citrus products were not readily available, British sailors suffered vitamin c deficiency that caused slow wound healing, tooth loss and eventual death due to the loss of ability to form collagen. Because vitamin C is the only antioxidant vitamin that can theoretically *both* prevent free radical damage to the skin *and* promote new collagen production in the skin, I suggest it for topical therapy using a serum that helps it penetrate through the superficial layers of the skin. Until more research data is out *proving* that these therapies make significant changes in sun damaged and aged skin, I do not suggest a lot of other topical anti-oxidant therapies as their combination can be extremely expensive. I have seen far too many women in their forties and fifties who have spent a few thousand dollars on these therapies who describe little if any improvement and are looking for a cosmetic facial surgical procedure. Save your money, with more time and more study physicians will be better able to advise their patients.

Pearl of Wisdom 18
There are no prospective, randomized double blinded studies that demonstrate that topical antioxidants such as Vitamin C either reduce or prevent skin aging.

It is a wonderful theory but proof is lacking.

Skin Care Products / Wrinkle Reversal

There are three classes of skin care products that improve the tightness of the skin and diminish fine lines and wrinkles. They are **Alpha** and **Beta Hydroxy Acids**, **Vitamin A Derivatives** (Retin-A, Renova and Retinol), and **DMAE** *(Table 2)*.

Skin Care Product Type	Examples	How They Work Theoretically	The Truth (Does It Work?)
Alpha and Beta Hydroxy Acids	Glycolic Acid Lactic Acid Salicylic Acid	Causes Superficial Layer of Skin to Shed, Increase Skin Collagen	Must have higher concentrations in products. Less than 8% little benefit. 8-15% very modest benefits. 20-30% most effective but not available over the counter.
Antioxidants	Vitamin C (Acsorbic Acid) Coenzyme Q10 Lipoic Acid Vitamin E Idebenone	Promotes Collagen Production and Neutralizes Free Radicals that Age Skin	Some are unstable compounds whose ability to penetrate the skin has not been proven. May be helpful but the jury is still out.
Vitamin A Derivatives	Retin-A Renova™ Retin A Micro™ Retinol	Increase Skin Cells, Thickens the Superficial and Deeper Layers of the Skin that Thin with Age.	All forms are proven effective except retinol. Retinol needs to be converted in skin to work, and how much this happens is questionable.
Dimethyaminoethanol	DMAE	Tightens Skin by Stabilizing Membranes	Noticeable but seldom dramatic improvement.

Table 2.

The Truth About Different Skin Care Products.

Alpha and Beta Hydroxy Acids (AHAs and BHAs) are proposed to tighten the skin surface and diminish fine lines and wrinkles. According to the FDA they can reduce wrinkles, spots and other signs of aging and sun damage. The more commonly used AHAs include glycolic acid, lactic acid, and ascorbic acid and the BHAs include salicylic acid (aspirin-like compound), and benzoic acid. The first reported case of use of AHAs was in ancient Egypt. Cleopatra used to take milk baths to add a certain glow to her legendary skin, and milk contains lactic acid. Alpha and Beta Hydroxy acids have been demonstrated to decrease the signs of aging by enhancing the shedding of the most superficial layer of the skin, the *epidermis*. Some claim that these compounds improve the quality of the *elastin fibers* and the collagen density of the middle layer of the skin, or *dermis* (see Chapter 2) thus reversing some of the deeper damage and sagging of the skin. Scientific evidence to support this claim is lacking.

Vitamin A Derivatives induce thickening of the epidermis, increase proliferation of skin cells, and act as a hormone to activate specific genes and proteins in the *dermal* layers. This hormonal activity increases deposition of new collagen in the *dermis*, reversing the thinning of this layer that occurs with age.

Pearl of Wisdom 19
The majority of Alpha and Beta hydroxy acids that are purchased in products from department stores are not present in sufficient concentration to make a difference worth footing the bill.

The effectiveness of an AHA skincare product depends mainly on the concentration of alpha hydroxy acids, not on the accompanying inactive ingredients with scientific-sounding names. The FDA regulates the concentration of these compounds that can be sold over the counter. For example, glycolic acid, one of the most popular AHAs, is sold in over the counter preparations at concentration less than one-fifth the concentration of AHAs that are found in preparations that physicians use (usually 5%). Products with alpha hydroxy acids in a concentration below 8% appear to be of no benefit. Most studies of 8-15% alpha hydroxy acids report very modest improvements in wrinkles and skin smoothness. When prescribed by a physician, the concentration is from 20% to 30%.

Topical Tretinoin (Retin-A) is the only form of vitamin A that has been studied and proven to accomplish these changes, and it must be prescribed by a doctor. In randomized, prospective, placebo controlled trials tretinoin was definitively proven to reduce fine lines and wrinkling, roughness and laxity of the skin. The key to success with Retin-A is: 1. It must be used at a minimum daily application concentration of .05% cream and 2. The results take about 6 months before they appear. The problem with this treatment is that it irritates the skin for the first 4 to 6 weeks, and most patients do not make it to the 6 month mark where the changes happen. Also most popular forms of tretinoin, which are less irritating, are at concentrations of .025% and .04% – not an adequate amount based on these important studies. Just like most things in life, no pain no gain, and when it comes to tretinoin therapy you must suffer the irritation during the initial phase of treatment to attain the benefits.

Pearl of Wisdom 20
Be aware that over the counter products contain the retinol form of vitamin A not tretinoin.

Retinol is not an effective form of vitamin A in the skin. It is not clear if the skin can convert retinol into enough retinoic acid (the active form), for the retinol products to have the same benefit as the prescription drug. The rate of conversion of retinol into retinoic acid is low, so a relatively large amount of retinol needs to be delivered into a cell to produce a significant effect. Most creams simply have too little retinol for that. For this reason, I do not recommend you buy any over the counter skin care products containing retinol, unless it is clear how much it contains.

DMAE is short for dimethylaminoethanol, a naturally occurring substance that facilitates the synthesis of a neurotransmitter acetylcholine. DMAE also may stimulate the synthesis of phosphatidylcholine, an important component of cell membranes. An intriguing finding in some DMAE studies was that it reduced the accumulation of lipofuscin deposits inside cells. Lipofuscin is a cellular pigment consisting of aggregated chunks of molecular waste. It tends to occur in the cells of older people. It is likely that lipofuscin is not simply a byproduct of aging but also contributes to the aging process.

The DMAE-skin connection is less researched. It has been demonstrated that DMAE causes some degree of skin tightening. However, despite speculation it remains unclear how DMAE firms the skin – whether by stabilizing the membranes, boosting acetylcholine, reducing lipofuscin deposits or none of the above. Whatever the mechanism, the effect of DMAE is often noticeable although seldom dramatic. Besides, even though DMAE can't fully reverse the existing facial sag, it may reduce the progression of facial sagging. Some people report a cumulative effect with continued use of DMAE.

A number of skin care companies released DMAE creams, most costing upward of $20 for a small jar. The prices reflect the hype and relative lack of competition from "supermarket" brands. DMAE itself is a rather simple substance, no more costly than alpha hydroxy acids or aspirin.

Chapter 10.
Quick Recovery Facial Plastic Surgery/
The Zen of Healing

Chapter 10.
Quick Recovery Facial Plastic Surgery/The Zen of Healing

There is a true art not only to how facial plastic surgery is performed, but also to how the surgeon modulates the healing process. This is the Zen of Healing. The rate at which patients heal after cosmetic surgery is dependent upon a number of factors, some of which the doctor and patient can control, and some they cannot. I have noticed in my practice that some patients will bruise and swell more than others with any trauma, and surgery is nothing more than precisely executed trauma to the facial tissues. I remember the case of a woman named Kathy who explained to me that if she bumped into a chair she would wind up with a grapefruit sized bruise on her leg. I can expect that patients like Kathy will require more intervention on my part to help minimize healing time.

Other than the minimally invasive techniques that are executed during a procedure, there are specific things that can be done before, during and after surgery that can minimize the untoward effects of surgery. As part of a holistic approach to healing, I implement traditional western medicine and homeopathic therapies to allow patients to enjoy a speedy recovery.

Before we begin to discuss the specifics of healing in the short term, it is important that all potential patients understand that healing is a process that must be monitored. There are different phases of healing that occur at days, weeks, and even months after surgery that must be followed by your surgeon. There are too many "hit and run" cosmetic surgical practices where 6 or 7 facelifts are performed every day – cutting corners to offer cheaper prices – and good long term post-operative care is not available. This approach results in longer healing time and poor results.

You can take control of your healing, even when your doctor does not. What follows is a guide for the patient. We will look at specific regimens that apply to resurfacing procedures (chemical peels and laser resurfacing) and others to more invasive surgical procedures.

Preparing for Surgery

All patients should have a complete physical examination by their internist (not their plastic surgeon) to assess their physical wellness and preparedness for surgery. A simple example is that poorly controlled high blood pressure can result in excessive bleeding after surgery and hence more bruising and swelling. Substitutions should be prescribed by your physician for any medications that will interact with anesthesia, thin the blood or inhibit surgical healing.

With this completed I start my patients on a strict regimen **two weeks prior to surgery.** The first thing patients must do is **avoid** medications, supplements, and habits that reduce the body's ability to stop bleeding and heal.

1) **Aspirin and Anti-inflammatories** (over the counter drugs such as Advil, Motrin, Aleve, Naproxen) impair platelet function necessary for clotting. Be aware that most cold remedies contain these drugs. Tylenol (acetominophen) is the only safe pain killer in the pre-operative period.

2) **Vitamin E** can thin the blood and cause more bleeding and bruising. Many health foods, shakes, and energy bars have excessive Vitamin E.

3) **Ginko Biloba** has an anti-coagulant affect and causes bleeding.

4) **Willow Bark** is an herbal supplement that contains salicin which is a precursor of aspirin.

5) **Smoking** increases swelling, limits blood flow to the skin during healing, and worsens scarring. If you smoke you need to refrain from smoking two weeks before and two weeks after surgery. That means no nicotine for 1 month, including no nicotine gums to curb cravings as nicotine is the culprit that affects healing. Due to the difficulty of abstaining from smoking, I often give patients a prescriptive medicine such as Wellbutrin™ that helps them kick the habit short term. There is a light at the end of the tunnel for smokers, as they can return to this destructive habit. What is wonderful is that patients will often stop smoking permanently after surgery; the surgery was the catalyst. There is a dual benefit in this situation. Not only are you healthier, but the surgical procedure will last longer in a non-smoker – about twice as long.

6) **Alcohol** intake should be avoided completely for 2 weeks before and 2 weeks after surgery as it also will thin the blood.

There are **dietary supplements that promote healing**, and these should be started 2 weeks before surgery.

1) **Vitamin C** is an essential co-factor for the production of collagen which is the glue that holds us together as we heal. I start all my patients on high dose Vitamin C therapy that includes 1000 milligrams taken three times a day. It should be taken with meals due to its acidic nature. Vitamin C is also a wonderful anti-oxidant that can minimize swelling in the post-operative healing.

2) **Arnica Montana** is an herb that grows wild in the Swiss Alps and has been used as a part of European herbal medicine for over a thousand years. It helps reduce bruising and swelling and shorten the recovery period after physical trauma. This means it helps speed healing, after a "planned trauma", plastic surgery. In one study, patients who wanted a facelift agreed to take either Arnica Montana or placebo, which was just a sugar pill without any medication in it. The comparison showed that the patients who took the placebo had on average 24% more bruising than the group that took Arnica Montana. On day seven after surgery, the patients who took the placebo had 41% more bruising than the patients who took Arnica Montana. I start all my patients 2 weeks before surgery on a form of this herb that dissolves under the tongue and readily gets into the bloodstream.

3) **Bromelain** is an anti-inflammatory formula containing the proteolytic enzyme from the stems of pineapples. Proteolytic enzymes are capable of dissolving proteins. They are most often used after sports injuries, to relieve edema, and after plastic surgical procedures to help with swelling. I usually prescribe 500 mg of Bromelain once a day. There are no controlled studies on this therapy, but I have used it in combination with Arnica Montana and have noticed a synergistic effect. Also, swelling has resolved 25% faster than with Arnica Montana alone.

4) **Valcyclovir** is an anti-herpes virus medication. Some patients have a tendency to get cold sores when they are stressed, and surgery is such a situation. I give 500 mg twice a day to prevent cold sore outbreaks in all surgeries if patients have this

predisposition. It is always a necessity when resurfacing the skin, as an outbreak in the skin with a laser resurfacing, chemical peel or dermabrasion can result in horrible scarring.

There are other "housekeeping" items to address within 2 weeks of surgery. For patients who color their hair, this should be done as close as possible to the date of surgery as the hair cannot be dyed again until 4 weeks after surgery. All medication should be purchased and at home before surgery. All post-operative instruction sheets should be reviewed and available at home to be referred to after surgery. **Do not eat after midnight the day before surgery** as it will delay the procedure. Finally, wear a comfortable outfit, usually a sweat suit, to surgery with a shirt that zips or buttons down the front so that it will not be necessary to pull it over the face after your procedure.

Post-Operative Care

There are treatments added immediately after surgery that help minimize the risk of complication and expedite healing. I continue patients on all the supplements they started two weeks before surgery, and add the following.

1) **Ice packs** will dramatically reduce swelling if applied for the first 24 hours after surgery. Frozen peas are ideal as they form fit to the face. A cloth should be placed over the face so that the ice pack is not directly on the skin, and cycles of 20 minutes on and 20 minutes off should be followed. This is extremely labor intensive. I often suggest that patients use my private duty nurses for this task. No matter how loving and committed a family member is, it is difficult for them to give you round the clock care. After 24 hours this therapy is not effective, but can be continued if it soothing.

2) **Elevation** of the head helps fluid to drain away from the face with gravity. During sleep the head should be on a minimum of three pillows. I usually suggest that this posture be maintained for a minimum of three weeks after surgery.

3) **Steroids** are strong anti-inflammatory medications that resist the body's ability to swell after trauma. I use methyprednisolone in a **Medrol Dose Pack**. There have been many studies in the plastic

surgical literature proving the efficacy of steroids. They can irritate the stomach, and cannot be used in diabetics. After resurfacing, steroid creams are used to help the pinkness resolve that will persist for 3 to 6 weeks.

4) **Antibiotics** are used as a prophylaxis to limit the possibility of infection after surgery. An infection will severely worsen the way incisions heal, and bad scars will result. Prevention is key.

5) **Polysporin Ointment** (triple antibiotic ointment) is extremely important in minimizing scarring. After the bandages are removed, the incision lines should be cleansed with hydrogen peroxide to remove crusting, and new ointment applied three times a day. Polysporin has been shown to improve the way scars heal when compared to other ointments (bacitracin and Neosporin alone) and so should always be used unless a patient has an allergy.

6) **Activity** must be limited for 2 weeks. Normal walking about the house is permitted immediately, and a short walk outside is fine after 48 hours. The head should not be brought below the level of the heart, and lifting over ten pounds should be avoided for two weeks. After two weeks you can increase activity slowly, and at the third week you can commence normal exercise. I have had patients who have developed delayed hematomas (blood collecting under the skin) or pulled incisions apart by returning to normal activity too quickly.

7) **Salty Foods** should be avoided as they cause fluid retention and swelling after surgery.

Scarring

Once the initial healing phase is over, after two weeks, the doctor and patient's work is not done. Incision lines must be cared for appropriately and monitored for scarring. The face **must be shielded from the sun.** Incision lines and resurfaced skin will turn brown if exposed. Even if you have a fraction of a hairline scar, if it is darker than the surrounding skin it will look like somebody drew on your face with a fine tip marker making the incisions extremely obvious. This does not simply mean applying a high SPF block (for example

SPF 50) to the skin, as UVA rays that change our pigmentation still penetrate. The face needs to be shielded from the sun with a large wide brimmed hat even when you are simply walking outside or driving in your car.

Incision lines will always scar to some degree, it is just a matter of how visibly and noticeably. Most times these scars are barely noticeable to the patient or surgeon. There is no such thing as surgery without a scar; if your doctor tells you this he/she is lying. Some procedures appear scarless because the incisions are hidden well. Incisions heal by the body producing collagen to seal them. They are usually pink and slightly raised for 4 to 6 weeks. They can be camouflaged with makeup during this time.

Sometimes collagen production is excessive causing a raised and obvious scar called a keloid. Some people are genetically predisposed to such scars, but they are aware from cuts and scratches over their lifetime. The way scars heal can be modulated by your surgeon as they evolve. I often have patients massage their incisions, which helps flatten scars and make them softer and more pliable. Massage should be done in moderation. I have had patients that get carried away, massage for half the day and cause inflammation and more scarring.

If scars start to worsen, there are treatments that can minimize scarring before it gets out of control. Steroid creams can be applied topically and silicone sheeting can be applied which helps soften the scar tissue and prevent scars from raising. When the problem is more severe a steroid called kenalog can be injected directly into the scar. When necessary this treatment can be repeated at intervals of 4 to 6 weeks.

Above all else be vigilant of your healing, take cues from your body, and keep your surgeon informed of all your concerns. As always an ounce of prevention is worth a pound of cure; correcting a problem as it evolves will lead to a happier result.

Even when the visible signs of surgery have resolved, the healing has just begun. The last 10% of swelling remains in the facial tissues and takes up to a total of 3 months to resolve. This will not be apparent to the outside observer, but is usually extremely obvious to patients. Residual numbness after surgery can exacerbate a patient's perception; just like after you go to the dentist, the numbness in your lip makes it feel as if it is three times normal size, but when you look in the mirror it is normal size.

Patients will often comment, "I don't look like myself." This is because normal facial expressions can also take 3 months' time to return, as the tightness and pulling of surgery resolve. I routinely hear from patients they look good at 6 weeks, look great at 3 months, and just when they thought they could not look any better look amazing at 6 months when everything has settled. All facial rejuvenative surgeries are a journey, and should be approached with this in mind.

Chapter 11.
Your Candidacy and
Choosing a Facial Plastic Surgeon

Chapter 11.
Your Candidacy and Choosing a Facial Plastic Surgeon

Where do we start when looking for a qualified facial plastic surgeon? On the internet? In a magazine or a phone book advertisement? Cosmetic surgery is more acceptable today than ever before, especially with the media's coverage of Botox and television shows such as *Extreme Makeover*. Unfortunately people are still secretive, and trying to get information about a good cosmetic surgeon or a good experience with a cosmetic procedure, even from friends, can be difficult.

The reason for caution is that any physician with a medical degree and a license to practice medicine can legally perform plastic surgery in the United States. This is why OB/GYN doctors are performing liposuction, laser skin resurfacing, and Botox in their offices, and dentists are performing rhinoplasties. I am amazed at all the local beauty salons on Long Island that offer collagen and Botox treatments without the presence of a physician!

Credentials are just the beginning when choosing a facial plastic surgeon. The public, in my opinion, is confused about this subject and with good reason. In today's competitive environment, in order to attract patients, it has been claimed that there exists only one board that certifies surgeons to perform plastic surgery. This is clearly not the case. There are five different legitimate boards that are either member boards of the American Board of Medical Specialties (ABMS) or equivalent boards. These boards include **The American Board of Facial Plastic and Reconstructive Surgery, The American Board of Plastic Surgery, The American Board of Dermatology, The American Board of Otolaryngology/Head and Neck Surgery,** and **The American Board of Ophthalmology.**

The American Board of Facial Plastic and Reconstructive Surgery certifies surgeons in the specific specialty area of plastic surgery of the face. The only surgeons who even qualify to take this specialists' board exam are either board certified diplomates of **The American**

Board of Otolaryngology/Head and Neck Surgery, or **The American Board of Plastic Surgery. The American Medical Association (AMA) recognizes The American Board of Otolaryngology/Head and Neck Surgery, The American Board of Plastic Surgery,** and **The American Board of Facial Plastic and Reconstructive Surgery** as legitimate certifying boards to test the qualifications of surgeons to perform facial plastic surgery.

Board Certified Plastic Surgeons complete three years of general surgery residency and 2 or 3 years of a plastic surgery residency. During the first three years of their training they perform colon resections, appendectomies, hemmorhoidectomies, gall bladder removals and thoracic and vascular surgery. During the 2 to 3 years in plastic surgery their time is divided amongst burn surgery, hand surgery, microsurgery, body reconstructive surgery, body cosmetic surgery, and finally facial plastic and reconstructive surgery. That is a tall bill to fill in only 2 or 3 years. Board certified and Fellowship Trained Facial Plastic Surgeons complete 5 years of an Otolaryngology/Head and Neck Surgery residency where they only operate on the face, nose, eyelids, head and neck first. During this time they perform cancer surgery for the head and neck, nose and face including reconstructive surgery on the face. They also perform cosmetic procedures such as rhinoplasty, eyelid lifting, and facelifting during this time. They then go on to complete an additional year of Fellowship training specializing further in the most updated techniques in Facial Plastic and Reconstructive Surgery. This Fellowship is sponsored by the American Academy of Facial Plastic and Reconstructive Surgery.

There are other associations and societies, different from boards, that are also highly credible. The **American Academy of Facial Plastic and Reconstructive Surgery (AAFPRS)** and the **American Society of Plastic Surgeons (ASPS),** are both highly credible organizations. They both require that their membership be board certified in their primary specialties, for the AAFPRS Board Certification in Head and Neck Surgery and the ASPS in Plastic Surgery.

You should also check your doctor's hospital affiliations. If a physician has privileges to perform surgery at an accredited hospital, this demonstrates that his or her performance and credentials are subject to regular scrutiny. While most plastic surgeons perform surgery only in their office, they do have privileges to perform surgery at a local hospital. If a doctor does not have these privileges, do not use that doctor.

Unfortunately, board certification is only the beginning to choosing your doctor. Board certification in Plastic Surgery or Facial Plastic Surgery means that your doctor has completed his or her residency training, passed rigorous comprehensive written and oral exams, and presented a series of surgical cases. But this does not mean he/she is a skilled surgeon; not all surgeons are created equal. Just as there are certain people who excel in sports due to their unique motor skills, there is a small percentage of

Pearl of Wisdom 21
When your Mercedes needs to be fixed, don't take it to the Ford dealer.

What I mean by this is that regardless of which of the above boards certify your surgeon, facial plastic surgery should be the only focus of the doctor's practice. The face is the most complex area of the entire body with respect to its anatomic relationships and nerves (the ones that move the face!) and it cannot be hidden with clothing. Your face is available for the entire world to see. Generalists or physicians who do all forms of body and face cosmetic surgery cannot do every operation perfectly; especially with the explosion of new technology and procedures it is almost impossible to keep up when only operating on the face, let alone the entire body. A good analogy would be to surgeons who only perform hip replacement surgery, and not the whole field of orthopedic surgery. When you perform a smaller scope of surgical procedures, your proficiency increases, the results improve, and the risk of complications decreases. Avoid the "Jack of all trades, master of none."

surgeons who have the ability to use their hands to sculpt tissue in an aesthetic way. What I am trying to say is that there are good surgeons and there are great surgeons, and to use our sports analogy, your job is to figure out who the pros are versus the minor leaguers.

How do you do this? Ask friends who have experience with a surgeon's work and ask your personal physician. Ask to see examples of the surgeon's work or talk to one or more patients about their surgical experience. Physicians who do the procedure you are interested in regularly, and do good work, will have an abundance of examples. Do not accept statements from your surgeon like... "my patients do not want me to show you their pictures" or "my patients are very private." This usually means that there are no examples of their work that they would want you to see. Most of my patients come from word-of-mouth referrals.

Pearl of Wisdom 22
There is no such medical specialty as Cosmetic Surgery.

There are many physicians from all backgrounds that join cosmetic surgical societies to learn how to perform procedures, but have no formal surgical training. If a doctor claims that he or she is a cosmetic surgeon, ask for more information about his or her formal medical training, surgical residency, and certifying board. The above noted boards certifying organizations should always be a part of your doctor's background.

Check out the surgeon's office and staff; be sure you will be treated the way you expect and that you feel comfortable there. Be sure the doctor is easy to talk to and is someone with whom you can relate. If you do not get along with your surgeon before surgery, do not expect things to get better after surgery.

Chapter 12:
Face to Face

Chapter 12:
Face to Face

FACE TO FACE is a humanitarian and educational surgical exchange program conducted under the auspices of the Educational and Research Foundation for the American Academy of Facial Plastic and Reconstructive Surgery (AAFPRS Foundation).

I am one of the surgeons who participate in this program, and I have dedicated a chapter of this book to ask for your support. Surgeons in FACE TO FACE assist those who suffer from facial deformities caused by congenital birth defects or by trauma. Most of those we have helped abroad have been children.

Unlike other programs, FACE TO FACE makes the educational exchange among facial plastic and reconstructive surgeons all over the world an integral part of its program. Our surgeons are men and women who believe that a more lasting impact is made on communities when our FACE TO FACE teams work together with local medical personnel to manage an individual's care. Mutual respect grows as different surgical approaches are discussed and demonstrated.

FACE TO FACE is staffed by medical personnel - facial plastic and reconstructive surgeons, nurses, speech pathologists and anesthesiologists - who donate their time and expertise, frequently for two weeks at a time. Members of the FACE TO FACE delegation have, for example, helped a two-year-old toddler in Russia abandoned by her parents at birth because of a congenital facial deformity. They have administered to a twelve-year old boy in a war zone in Croatia where he sustained severe facial trauma after playing with a loaded rifle. And they have cared for women and children in this country where domestic violence has wreaked havoc on their lives both emotionally and physically. These are faces that you have seen on the news and sometimes in your own community. With domestic violence victims, after they leave the abusive relationship, the scars and deformities of their faces are a constant and lasting reminder of their past; removing them helps people move on to lead happier and more successful lives.

I am extremely blessed in being able to help these women. I perform pro-bono reconstructive surgery on approximately a dozen survivors of domestic violence a year. Let me tell you a story about one of my patients, Melissa. Melissa had been beaten for so long that her face literally collapsed.

Her nose, after 17 years of punches by her abuser, had flattened flush against her face, making it difficult for her to breathe. The repeated blows had caused the tendons to loosen from her lower eyelids, which then drooped – a condition more common to people in their 70s than to a woman who is 42.

In a six-hour operation I harvested a rectangular piece of bone from her skull, reshaped it, and used it to rebuild the bridge of Melissa's nose. I used cartilage from her right ear to shape the nose's tip. Finally, I made incisions under her eyes to lift the sagging lids.

Melissa said getting surgery was never something she considered because of its high cost. "There was always something more important that my kids needed," she said. Now, she said, "I can look in the mirror without that constant reminder."

Melissa suffered for years at the hands of her partner, who often aimed his blows at her face. "When I'm done with you, no one else will ever want you," she remembers him threatening.

I have been donating my services to domestic violence victims for about seven years, ever since I performed facial surgery on a woman who initially told me she had been in an auto accident. I discovered she was a victim of domestic abuse when she returned a few months later. My work had been completely destroyed.

The FACE TO FACE program both in the United States and abroad offers individuals the opportunity to overcome the physical limitations placed on them by circumstances beyond their control – deformities at birth, domestic violence and war. Our surgeons use their expertise to perform plastic and reconstructive surgery of the face, head, and neck. This includes the following procedures: cleft lip and cleft palate repair; microtia reconstruction – the surgical creation of external ears for infants born without them; rebuilding of all forms of congenital facial and cranial deformities; reconstruction of facial soft tissues after war injuries, burns, domestic violence and cancer excisions; the excision of childhood facial tumors and reconstruction. While the patients still have enormous hurdles to overcome, at least they are given a chance to deal with them without physical limitations.

We are very proud of our humanitarian programs and how they are changing lives for the better. The American Society of Association Executives (ASAE) honored AAFPRS with the 1995 Summit Award for FACE TO FACE: The National Domestic Violence Project and the 1995 Award of Excellence for FACE TO FACE: International. The American Medical Association Board of Trustees has given the AAFPRS the 1995 President's Citation for Service to the Public Award.

FACE TO FACE depends on people like you to make a difference. Although surgeons and other medical personnel give freely of their time and expertise, FACE TO FACE still needs funding to cover ancillary expenses. We always appreciate donations of medical supplies and equipment, but when one of our international colleagues is in urgent need of equipment we provide the funding for the purchase. We also need funds to offset costs for developing teaching symposia and producing educational materials.

Because the Educational and Research Foundation for the American Academy of Facial Plastic and Reconstructive Surgery is a non-profit organization (a 501 (c)(3)), your contribution to FACE TO FACE is tax deductible to the fullest extent provided by law. Your gift now can change the lives of thousands – of men, women and children, both here at home and abroad.

For those of you who live in the tri-state area, I hold a benefit on Long Island in October every year. It is a wonderful night of music, entertainment, cocktails, food and dancing with the proceeds going to the FACE TO FACE Organization to further our cause. I hope to see you there and shake your hand and thank you for your support! For more information please do not hesitate to contact my office at:

900 Northern Boulevard, Suite 130

Great Neck, New York 11021

(516)773-4646

www.newyorkfacialplasticsurgery.com

Index

**The New York Center for
Facial Plastic and Laser Surgery**
900 Northern Boulevard
Suite 130
Great Neck, NY 11021
(516) 773-4646
www.newyorkfacialplasticsurgery.com

**American Academy of Facial
Plastic and Reconstructive Surgery**
310 S. Henry Street
Alexandria, VA 22314
(703) 299-9291
www.aafprs.org

**American Board of Facial Plastic
and Reconstructive Surgery**
115C South St. Asaph Street
Alexandria, VA 22314
(703) 549-3223
www.abfprs.org

**American Society of Plastic and
Reconstructive Surgeons**
444 East Algonquin Road
Arlington Heights, IL 60005-4664
www.plasticsurgery.org
(847) 228-9900

American Board of Plastic Surgery
Seven Penn Center, Suite 400
1635 Market Street
Philadelphia, PA 19103-2204
(215)587-9322
www.abplsurg.org

American Academy of Dermatology
1350 I St. NW, Suite 870
Washington, DC 20005-4355
(202) 842-3555
www.aad.org

American Board of Otolaryngology/Head and Neck Surgery
5615 Kirby Drive
Suite 600
Houston, TX 77005
(713) 850-1104
www.aboto.org

American Board of Medical Specialties
1007 Church Street
Suite 404
Evanston, IL 60201-5913
(847) 491-9091
www.abms.org

American Board of Ophthalmology
111 Presidential Boulevard, Suite 241
Bala Cynwyd, PA 19004-1075
(610) 664-1175
www.abop.org

The American Society for Aesthetic Plastic Surgery
www.surgery.org
1-800-ASAPS11

Restylane
www.restylaneusa.com
Medicis

Botox Cosmetic
www.botoxcosmetic.com
Allergan

Radiesse
www.radiesse.com
BioForm Medical

FACE TO FACE
www.facetofacesurgery.org

Inamed Aesthetics:
    Captique
    Cosmoderm
    Cosmoplast
    Zyderm
    Zyplast
    Hylaform
www.inamed.com

AlloDerm
www.lifecell.com

Thermage
www.thermage.com

Contour Threadlift
www.contourthreads.com

OBAGI
www.obagi.com

www.rhinoplastyexpert.com

NOTES

NOTES

NOTES

NOTES

NOTES

NOTES

NOTES

NOTES

NOTES

NOTES

NOTES

NOTES

NOTES

NOTES

NOTES